Curbside Consultation
in Cataract Surgery

49 Clinical Questions

CURBSIDE CONSULTATION IN OPHTHALMOLOGY
SERIES

SERIES EDITOR, DAVID F. CHANG, MD

Curbside Consultation
in Cataract Surgery

49 Clinical Questions

Editor

David F. Chang, MD
Clinical Professor
University of California
San Francisco, California
Altos Eye Physicians
Los Altos, California

Associate Editors

Terry Kim, MD
Associate Professor of Ophthalmology
Duke University School of Medicine
Director of Fellowship Programs
Associate Director, Cornea and Refractive Surgery
Duke University Eye Center
Durham, North Carolina

Thomas A. Oetting, MS, MD
Clinical Associate Professor of Ophthalmology
University of Iowa
Department of Ophthalmology and Visual Sciences
Iowa City, Iowa

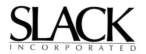

SLACK
INCORPORATED

*Delivering the best in health care information
and education worldwide*

www.slackbooks.com

ISBN: 978-1-55642-799-2

Copyright © 2007 by SLACK Incorporated

Contact SLACK Incorporated for more information about other books in this field or about the availability of our books from distributors outside the United States.

Published by: SLACK Incorporated
6900 Grove Road
Thorofare, NJ 08086 USA
Telephone: 856-848-1000
Fax: 856-853-5991
www.slackbooks.com

Curbside consultation in cataract surgery / editor, David F. Chang ; associate editors, Terry Kim, Thomas A. Oetting.
p. ; cm. -- (Curbside consultation in ophthalmology series)
Includes bibliographical references and index.
ISBN-13: 978-1-55642-799-2 (alk. paper)
ISBN-10: 1-55642-799-9 (alk. paper)
1. Cataract--Surgery--Miscellanea. I. Kim, Terry. II. Oetting, Thomas A. III. Series.
[DNLM: 1. Cataract Extraction--Handbooks. WW 39 C975 2007]

RE451.C87 2007
617.7'42059--dc22
2006100223

Contents

Dedication

We all owe much of our success to the help of key individuals who took a personal interest in our growth, education, and development. When I started this book project in early 2006, I had just spoken at the memorials for two of my most important mentors. Doing so reminded me of how truly fortunate I am to have had their inspiration and guidance during my formative years.

Steven G. Kramer, MD, PhD was the Chief of Ophthalmology at the University of California, San Francisco (UCSF) for 27 years. His tenure began in 1975 when, at the age of 34, he became the youngest ophthalmology chair in the country. Although Steve was an accomplished research scientist and gifted corneal surgeon, his personal career became secondary to the stewardship of a premier ophthalmology department. He recruited and nurtured a full-time faculty that grew from 2 members to 16 members during his tenure. He championed an ophthalmic basic science department that often led the nation in National Institutes of Health (NIH) grants, and in 1988 realized the dream of combining both basic and clinical sciences under the same roof of a newly constructed, state-of-the-art eye center.

Steve's greatest accomplishment was developing a residency program that was for many years the most requested in the national residency match. He made resident education the department's priority and restricted fellowships at UCSF so that fellows would not compete for surgical cases and faculty attention. Steve sought to personally mentor each of us and as a result, he was not only our chief but also our friend. He performed magic tricks (his hobby) at Grand Rounds, was our department's softball captain and pitcher, and insisted that we always call him "Steve." UCSF became the epitome of a "residents' program," and the many outstanding ophthalmologists who trained under him are Steve Kramer's greatest legacy.

My mother, Carol Chang, was born and raised in Shanghai, China. Upon graduating college in 1947, she won a prestigious government award to study abroad. Throughout its long history, China had always struggled to feed its population. As an idealistic and patriotic young woman, my mother's ambition was to develop novel ways to improve her country's nutrition. Toward this end, she earned her Biochemistry PhD from Cornell with a research interest in nutrition. Sadly, like many other overseas Chinese students, she could not return to China following the Communist takeover. For many years, the Cultural Revolution precluded any communication with her family and it would be 30 years before she was able to visit China in 1977 to see them again. Pursuing her education abroad had unexpectedly cost my mother her country, her professional goal, and all contact with her family. Mom's ultimate sacrifice, however, was giving up that hard-earned career to raise her 2 children full-time and to navigate the many challenges that all immigrant parents face. She managed to rear and mentor not one, but 2 ophthalmologists in the process. My sister, Lisa, followed me through the UCSF residency and enjoyed Steve Kramer's guidance and support as well.

It is with respect and appreciation that I dedicate this book to mentors everywhere, and in loving memory of Steven Kramer and Carol Chang.

David F. Chang, MD

To my wife, Ellie, and my children, Ashley and Kayley, for their never ending love, support, and understanding.

To all my resident and fellow trainees, who constantly stimulate my mind and inspire me to be a better teacher.

To all of my mentors, for their advice and guidance throughout my career.

Terry Kim, MD

I dedicate this book to my understanding family who have made life so much fun: my wife, Marguerite, and my children, Drew, Lilli, and Blake. I have learned so much from the many residents who have passed through our training program at the University of Iowa and am fortunate to count them now as my good friends. Finally, I join David and Terry in dedicating this book to my mentors who have helped me to grow over the years.

Thomas A. Oetting, MS, MD

Acknowledgments

Organizing, editing, and producing any textbook is hard work, but we have enjoyed the creative process of introducing a new and hopefully interesting educational format. We would like to acknowledge the many people who helped us develop this book. Foremost, we applaud the efforts of our chapter authors. Despite their very busy speaking and writing schedules, they were able to find the time to do one more task. They took on their questions with enthusiasm and stayed on schedule.

In order to ensure that we posed pertinent questions, we first tested them on a panel of residents and busy clinicians in both private practice and academics. We greatly appreciate the efforts of the following surgeons who critiqued our list of potential questions: Rosa Braga-Mele, Geoffrey Broocker, Bonnie Henderson, Tim Johnson, Ed Kim, Donna Lee, Scott Lee, Jeff Maassen, Hunter Newsom, Erin O'Malley, Luis Omphroy, Steve Sauer, Pulin Shah, Andrew Sorenson, George Yang, and Sonia Yoo.

We are indebted to the fine team at SLACK Incorporated's Health Care Books and Journals Division for their guidance and help in making this textbook idea become a reality. Jennifer Briggs and John Bond helped us to organize the project and kept us on task. April Billick oversaw the layout and the editing process with much help from Kimberly Shigo. It was a privilege working with such an experienced and dedicated group of professionals. We would also like to thank Laura Pitlick for her help with editing and scheduling.

Finally, we would like to thank our families for allowing us to devote our time and energy toward completing yet "one more project."

David F. Chang, MD
Terry Kim, MD
Thomas A. Oetting, MS, MD

About the Editor

David F. Chang, MD is a Summa Cum Laude graduate of Harvard College and earned his MD at Harvard Medical School. He completed his ophthalmology residency at the University of California, San Francisco (UCSF) where he is now a clinical professor. Dr. Chang is Chairman of the American Academy of Ophthalmology (AAO) Annual Meeting Program Committee, having previously chaired the Cataract Program Subcommittee. He organized and was the program co-chair for the first 6 AAO "Spotlight on Cataracts" Symposia.

He has been selected to deliver the following named lectures: Transamerica Lecture (UCSF), Williams Lecture (UCSF), Wolfe Lecture (University of Iowa), DeVoe Lecture (Columbia-Harkness), Gettes Lecture (Wills Eye Hospital), Helen Keller Lecture (University of Alabama), Kayes Lecture (University of Washington, St. Louis), and Thorpe Lecture (Pittsburgh Ophthalmology Society). He has received 2 AAO Secretariat Awards (2003 and 2006). He was the inaugural recipient of the UCSF Department of Ophthalmology's Distinguished Alumni Award (2005) and received the 2006 Charlotte Baer Award honoring the outstanding clinical faculty member (of more than 2000 active clinical faculty) at the UCSF Medical School. He was the 2007 recipient of the Strampelli Medal from the Italian Ophthalmological Society.

Dr. Chang is vice-chair of the AAO Practicing Ophthalmologist Curriculum Committee for Cataract and Anterior Segment, which developed the American Board of Ophthalmology knowledge base for the MOC examination. He is also on the AAO Cataract Preferred Practice Pattern Panel. Dr. Chang is chair of the American Society of Cataract and Refractive Surgery (ASCRS) Cataract Clinical Committee and is a member of the ASCRS Eye Surgery Education Council Presbyopia Task Force. He is on the scientific advisory board for the UCSF Collaborative Vision Research Group, American Medical Optics, Calhoun Vision, Medennium, Peak Surgical, and Visiogen, and is the medical monitor for the Visiogen Synchrony accommodating IOL Food and Drug Administration (FDA) monitored trial. He is co-chief medical editor for *Cataract & Refractive Surgery Today* and is the cataract editor for 2 online educational sites: the AAO's "Specialty Clinical Updates" and the *Ocular Surgery News* "Ophthalmic Hyperguides." He is editor of the *Cataract & Refractive Surgery Today Virtual Textbook of Cataract Surgery* and was the principal author of *Phaco Chop: Mastering Techniques, Optimizing Technology, and Avoiding Complications* (published by SLACK Incorporated), which was the first ophthalmic textbook to have a paired DVD featuring instructional surgical video.

About the Associate Editors

Terry Kim, MD received his medical degree from Duke University School of Medicine and completed his residency and chief residency in ophthalmology at Emory Eye Center. He continued with his fellowship training in Cornea and External Disease and Refractive Surgery at Wills Eye Hospital. He was then recruited to Duke University Eye Center, where he serves as principal investigator on a major research grant from the National Eye Institute to investigate innovative corneal adhesives. Dr. Kim was formerly the Director of the Residency Program and now serves as the Director of Fellowship Programs.

Dr. Kim's academic accomplishments include his extensive publications in the peer-reviewed literature, which include close to 100 journal articles and textbook chapters. He is also co-author and co-editor of a comprehensive textbook on corneal diseases and surgery, entitled *The Requisites in Ophthalmology: Anterior Segment*. Dr. Kim has delivered over 100 invited lectures both nationally and internationally. His clinical and research work has earned him honors and grants from the American Academy of Ophthalmology (AAO), American Society of Cataract and Refractive Surgery (ASCRS), National Institutes of Health, Fight for Sight/Research to Prevent Blindness, Heed Ophthalmic Foundation, Alcon Laboratories, and Allergan. He is also listed in *Best Doctors in America, Best Doctors in North Carolina, and America's Top Ophthalmologists*. Dr. Kim is on the Annual Program Committee for AAO and on the Cornea Clinical Committee for ASCRS. He serves as consultant to the Ophthalmic Devices Panel of the FDA and sits on the Editorial Board for the journals *Cornea, Cataract & Refractive Surgery Today*, and *Review of Ophthalmology*.

Thomas A. Oetting, MS, MD is an Associate Professor and the Residency Program Director in the Ophthalmology Department at the University of Iowa. He also serves as Chief of Ophthalmology and Deputy Director for Surgery for the Iowa City VAMC. He received a Bachelor's degree in Electrical Engineering, Master's degree in Biomedical Engineering, and a doctor of medicine degree from Duke University. He did his residency in ophthalmology at the University of Iowa. While a faculty member at Iowa, he won the Resident Teaching Award in 2000, 2001, 2002, and 2005. He co-founded the eyerounds.com Web site at the University of Iowa, which provides a rich source of material for ophthalmologists.

Dr. Oetting has been an active educator nationally. He has served on the AAO annual meeting cataract subcommittee and practicing ophthalmology curriculum for the past 3 years. He has published extensively on resident education and has taught courses in this area at the AAO, the ASCRS, and as a visiting professor. Dr Oetting has been the editor for the award winning "Morning Rounds" section for the *AAO EyeNet* magazine for the past 8 years. He was awarded the AAO Secretariat and Achievement Awards for these efforts. His electronic book *Cataract Surgery for Greenhorns* is a popular source for resident eye surgeons. He has been an invited lecturer at the Harvard and Madison Phacoemulsification Courses and the Lancaster Course. He has written numerous articles on eye surgery and is a reviewer for several journals including the *Journal of Cataract and Refractive Surgery* and *Archives of Ophthalmology*.

Contributing Authors

Iqbal Ike K. Ahmed, MD, FRCSC
Credit Valley Hospital
Mississauga, Ontario, Canada

Lisa B. Arbisser, MD
Cofounder, Eye Surgeons Associates PC,
Iowa and Illinois Quad Cities
Clinical Adjunct Associate Professor
University of Utah
John A. Moran Eye Center
Salt Lake City, Utah

Steve A. Arshinoff, MD, FRCSC
York Finch Eye Associates
Humber River Regional Hospital
The University of Toronto
Toronto, Ontario, Canada

Rosa Braga-Mele, MEd, MD, FRCSC
Associate Professor
University of Toronto, Canada
Director of Cataract Unit and Surgical
Teaching
Mt. Sinai Hospital, Toronto
Toronto, Ontario, Canada

Scott E. Burk, MD, PhD
Cincinnati Eye Institute
Cincinnati, Ohio

Stanley Chang, MD
Department of Ophthalmology
Columbia University
Edward Harkness Eye Institute
New York, New York

Robert J. Cionni, MD
Cincinnati Eye Institute
Cincinnati, Ohio

Garry P. Condon, MD
Drexel University College of Medicine
Department of Ophthalmology
Allegheny General Hospital
Pittsburgh, Pa

Alan S. Crandall, MD
Department of Ophthalmology
University of Utah
John A. Moran Eye Center
Salt Lake City, Utah

Elizabeth A. Davis, MD, FACS
Minnesota Eye Consultants, PA
Bloomington, Minn

Eric D. Donnenfeld, MD
Ophthalmic Consultants of Long Island
Rockville Centre, NY

I. Howard Fine, MD
Drs. Fine, Hoffman & Packer, LLC
Oregon Eye Institute
Eugene, Ore

William J. Fishkind, MD, FACS
Co-Director
Fishkind & Bakewell Eye Care and Surgery
Center
Tucson, Ariz
Clinical Professor
University of Utah
Salt Lake City, Utah
Clinical Instructor
University of Arizona
Tucson, Ariz

Luther L. Fry, MD
Clinical Assistant Professor
Department of Ophthalmology
University of Kansas Medical Center
Kansas City, Kan

Johnny Gayton, MD
Eyesight Associates of Middle Georgia
Warner Robins, Ga

James P. Gills, MD
St. Luke's Cataract & Laser Institute
Tarpon Springs, Fla

Howard V. Gimbel, MD, MPH, FRCSC, FACS
Gimbel Eye Center
Calgary, Alberta, Canada

Bonnie An Henderson, MD
Ophthalmic Consultants of Boston
Harvard Medical School
Boston, Mass

Warren E. Hill, MD, FACS
East Valley Ophthalmology
Mesa, Ariz

Jack T. Holladay, MD, MSEE, FACS
Clinical Professor of Ophthalmology
Baylor College of Medicine
Houston, Tex

Douglas D. Koch, MD
Professor and the Allen, Mosbacher, and
Law Chair in Ophthalmology
Cullen Eye Institute
Baylor College of Medicine
Houston, Tex

Paul Koch, MD
Koch Eye Associates
Warwick, RI

Manus C. Kraff, MD
Professor of Clinical Ophthalmology
Northwestern University
Chicago, Ill

Stephen Lane, MD
Adjunct Professor
University of Minnesota
Stillwater, Minn

Richard A. Lewis, MD
Consultant
Grutzmacher and Lewis
Sacramento, Calif

Richard L. Lindstrom, MD
Minnesota Eye Consultants, PA
Minneapolis, Minn

Richard J. Mackool, MD
Director
Mackool Eye Institute
Astoria, NY
Clinical Professor
New York University
New York, NY
Attending Surgeon
New York Eye and Ear Infirmary
New York, NY

Francis S. Mah, MD
Assistant Professor, Department of
Ophthalmology
University of Pittsburgh School of
Medicine
Medical Co-Director
The Charles T. Campbell Ophthalmic
Mi-crobiology Laboratory
Cornea, External Diseases, and Refractive
Surgery Service
UPMC Eye Center
Assistant Professor, Department of
Pathology
University of Pittsburgh School of
Medicine
Pittsburg, Pa

Nick Mamalis, MD
University of Utah
Department of Ophthalmology
John A. Moran Eye Center
Salt Lake City, Utah

Samuel F. Masket, MD
Advanced Vision Care
Los Angeles, Calif

Kevin M. Miller, MD
Jules Stein Eye Institute
Department of Ophthalmology
David Getten School of Medicine at UCLA
Los Angeles, Calif

Louis D. "Skip" Nichamin, MD
Laurel Eye Clinic, LLP
Brookville, Pa

Randall J. Olson, MD
The John A. Moran Presidential Professor
and Chair of Ophthalmology and Visual
Sciences
Director
John A. Moran Eye Center
University of Utah Health Sciences Center
Salt Lake City, Utah

Robert H. Osher, MD
Professor of Ophthalmology
University of Cincinnati
Medical Director Emeritus
Cincinnati Eye Institute
Cincinnati, Ohio

Mark Packer, MD
Drs. Fine, Hoffman & Packer, LLC
Eugene, Ore

Francis W. Price, Jr, MD
Medical Director
Price Vision Group
President—Board of Directors
Cornea Research Foundation of America
Indianapolis, Ind

Michael B. Raizman, MD
Ophthalmic Consultants of Boston
Director, Cornea and Cataract Service
New England Eye Center
Associate Professor of Ophthalmology
Tufts University School of Medicine
Boston, Mass

Kenneth J. Rosenthal, MD, FACS
Surgeon Director
Rosenthal Eye & Facial Plastic Surgery
Great Neck, NY
Associate Professor of Ophthalmology
John A. Moran Eye Center
Univeristy of Utah Health Sciences Center
Salt Lake City, Utah
Assistant Professor of Ophthalmology
New York University Medical School
New York, NY

Thomas Samuelson, MD
Attending Surgeon
Minnesota Eye Consultants and Phillips
Eye Institute
Adjunct Associate Professor
University of Minnesota
Minneapolis, Minn

Barry S. Seibel, MD
Seibel Vision Surgery
Los Angeles, Calif

Bradford J. Shingleton, MD
Ophthalmic Consultants of Boston
Boston, Mass

Kerry D. Solomon, MD
Director of Cornea, Cataract and Refractive
Surgery
Storm Eye Institute
Medical Director
Magill Laser Center
Director
Magill Research Center
Charleston, SC

Walter J. Stark, MD
Boone Pickens Professor of Ophthalmology
The Director of the Stark-Mosher Center for
Cataract and Corneal Services
The Wilmer Eye Institute
The Johns Hopkins Hospital
Baltimore, Md

Roger F. Steinert, MD
Department of Ophthalmology
University of California at Irvine
Irvine, Calif

R. Bruce Wallace III, MD, FACS
Wallace Eye Surgery
Alexandria, La

Kevin L. Waltz, OD, MD
Eye Surgeons of Indiana
Indianapolis, Ind

Preface

The informal "curbside consult" is a commonplace occurrence in every field of medicine. This is where a busy clinician, when faced with a diagnostic or treatment dilemma, solicits practical advice from a knowledgeable expert. Every day, these brief consultations take place in clinic hallways, over the telephone, and by email. The question is brief and concise. The advice is practical, to the point, and based upon that expert's knowledge, judgment, and experience.

This textbook on cataract techniques seeks to provide a compendium of this information—answers to the thorny questions most commonly posed to specialists by practicing colleagues. This educational question-and-answer format is unique among other publications. Just as a curbside consult is distinguished from a lecture or an instruction course, so is this compilation different from a scientific journal or standard textbook. Most of these clinical questions do not individually merit a lecture, review article, or book chapter. In most cases, these questions are not answered definitively by the scientific literature.

The questions were compiled by my associate editors and myself and then posed to 49 of the top cataract consultants in North America. We have divided the book into 3 sections: preoperative, intraoperative, and postoperative questions. The advice from our surgical consultants is based upon personal experience, their review of the evidence-based literature, and in some cases, their own clinical studies. I asked that our consultants' answers meet my 4 criteria of content—the 4 "Cs." The advice must be current (timely), concise (summarizing), credible (evidence based), and clinically relevant (practical).

As you read, imagine that you have tracked down and then posed your question to a leading authority by email, telephone, or in person. Whether you read the book from cover to cover, read 1 question at a time (whenever your schedule allows), or simply employ this as a handy reference for when difficult problems arise, I hope that you will find this novel educational format to be both stimulating and useful.

David F. Chang, MD

Foreword

We ophthalmologists are frequently confronted with patients who represent unusual challenges, and in preparation for those cases, we may consult the literature, surgical atlases, and textbooks. However, most commonly, we call friends, colleagues, associates, or recognized experts in the particular area of challenge. Certainly, the faculty at major meetings are always confronted following their session with ophthalmologists who come to ask questions about one of their patients who present a unique challenge.

In this book, David F. Chang, MD has brought together recognized experts in cataract surgery and has given each of them a specific problem to address. The book is appropriately organized into 3 sections: preoperative, intraoperative, and postoperative questions. Each of the questions focuses on a highly specific problem. The authors are all well known and highly recognized for their ability to manage that particular problem and each author describes exactly how he or she handles that situation. The questions are precisely focused and appropriate without being exhaustive or overburdened with caveats. This is a very easily readable and interesting book. The concise nature of each of the questions allows for continuous reading; however, it will probably find its greater utilization as a reference source as surgeons return to the book to deal with a specific problem when it arises.

Dr. Chang is an internationally recognized surgeon, teacher, researcher, author, and clinician. It was a brilliant insight to recognize that there is a need for the book, and we are fortunate that he has organized the topics and brought together the faculty to address that need within our resource material. This is a book that will be helpful to every surgeon, from the novice to the expert, and will find its place among the most commonly referred-to sources by anterior segment surgeons.

I. Howard Fine, MD
Drs. Fine, Hoffman & Packer, LLC
Oregon Eye Institute
Eugene, Ore

SECTION I

PREOPERATIVE QUESTIONS

WITH COEXISTING MACULAR DISEASE, HOW CAN I TELL WHETHER IT IS WORTH DOING CATARACT SURGERY?

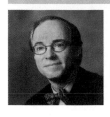

Douglas D. Koch, MD

Cataracts and macular changes often coexist. As clinicians, we frequently must estimate the potential clinical benefit of cataract surgery and educate the patient regarding reasonable expectations for postoperative visual acuity. Fortunately, a number of modalities are available to assist in this process. The goal is to estimate cataract density, current macular function, and macular changes that could occur as a result of cataract surgery.

Clinical Evaluation

The clinical history can often be informative. What type of visual loss is present? Complaints such as distorted vision or blind spots in vision suggest primarily a macular etiology. If there has been slow, progressive loss of vision, particularly accompanied by selected visual complaints (eg, "can't see to drive at night but reading is OK"), then the cataract is implicated as the overriding problem.

The examination process should include a detailed refraction for distance and near visual acuity, Amsler grid testing, and slit-lamp and fundus examinations as well as other possible tests. These might include retinoscopy to evaluate the quality of the red reflex and visualization of the macula with a 78-D or 90-D lens, Hruby lens, or even a direct ophthalmoscope. If the red reflex is relatively clear and the macula can be visualized, then it is unlikely that lens opacity is a major cause of visual loss.

Clinical examination can also include an estimation of the quality of the patient's fixation. Image a thin, short slit beam on the patient's fovea. Ask the patient to look at the top, bottom, and finally the center of the light. Assess the quality of the patient's fixation during these steps and ask the patient to describe the quality of the image. Is fixation crisp or uncertain and unsteady? Is the slit beam seen as uniform or are portions missing? Unfortunately, some patients are not able to perform this test (especially the description of the slit beam). In these situations, comparison with the patient's performance in the fellow eye is sometimes helpful.

In most patients with cataracts and macular abnormalities, this is all that is required. Patients who might benefit from additional testing include those with active vascular disease (eg, diabetic retinopathy), epiretinal membranes, and advanced cataracts that preclude adequate visualization of the macula.

Supplemental Preoperative Tests of Visual Function

Additional subjective and objective tests are available for evaluating macular function. Unfortunately, they tend to underestimate visual potential and hence are often least helpful in the very patients in whom it is most difficult to make a clinical assessment (ie, patients with advanced cataracts). Available tests include the Guyton-Minkowski potential acuity meter (PAM) (Mentor, Norwell, Mass), laser interferometer, and scanning laser ophthalmoscope. In recent years, there has been growing evidence that tests of near acuity with a brightly illuminated near card may be among the most accurate approaches. These techniques include the potential acuity pinhole[1] in which a 1.0-mm pinhole is placed over the patient's glasses while illuminating the card with a Finoff transilluminator, measurement of near vision with a +8.0-D lens and bright illumination of the near card,[2] and use of an illuminated near card device.[3] Interestingly, these near-vision tests are helpful variants of the simple comparison of best-corrected distance and near visual acuities.

From a practical standpoint, I rarely use these ancillary tests of visual acuity. In general, if the cataract is sufficiently severe to preclude adequate visualization of the macula and assessment of its function, then surgery at a minimum facilitates monitoring of retinal status and often noticeably improves the patient's peripheral vision.

There are, however, 2 objective tests that are sometimes invaluable for evaluating macular structure and vascular integrity. Optical coherence tomography (OCT) is often extremely helpful in patients with epiretinal membranes and/or possible macular edema or other macular pathology (Figures 1-1 and 1-2). If the OCT shows macular thickening or evidence of vitreomacular traction, then I usually refer to a vitreoretinal surgeon for evaluation prior to performing cataract surgery.

Likewise, fluorescein angiography can be helpful to evaluate active vascular leakage or macular ischemia. Again, preoperative retinal consultation may be helpful.

Informed Consent

To help the patient form realistic expectations, it is important to provide your best estimate of postoperative acuity and to emphasize the uncertainty of your estimation.

The clinician must also discuss the potential impact of cataract surgery on postoperative macular function. For eyes with age-related macular degeneration, preliminary

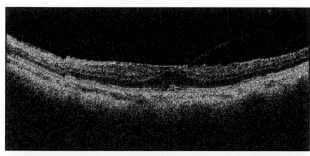

Figure 1-1. OCT image of left macula of patient with symmetrical 2+ nuclear sclerotic cataracts but asymmetrical visual acuities of 20/25 and 20/50. There is an epiretinal membrane with vitreous traction and macular edema. Cataract surgery was deferred.

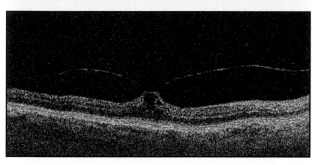

Figure 1-2. OCT showing a stage 1 macular hole. In this instance, the vitreoretinal surgeon recommended cataract surgery to precipitate a posterior vitreous detachment. This occurred postoperatively, and the patient regained vision of 20/25.

evidence from the Age-Related Eye Disease Study (AREDS) suggests that cataract surgery does not exacerbate macular disease (Frederick L. Ferris, personal communication, July 2006). However, there is still some controversy about this. Certainly, patients with epiretinal membranes and macular retinal vascular disease (eg, diabetic retinopathy) are at risk for increased edema postoperatively. They may be resistant to medical therapy and may require more invasive measures such as intravitreal injection of corticosteroids, laser coagulation of incompetent vessels, and pars plana vitrectomy. In some instances, postoperative macular edema is recalcitrant to all forms of therapy.

Conclusion

These patients are a true test of the cataract surgeon's clinical acumen. Despite the plethora of means for evaluating these eyes, it is not always possible to accurately predict the postoperative outcome. Candid and detailed informed consent is essential in assisting patients afflicted with this frightening problem.

References

1. Melki SA, Safar A, Martin J, Ivanova A, Adi M. Potential acuity pinhole: a simple method to measure potential visual acuity in patients with cataracts, comparison to potential acuity meter. *Ophthalmology*. 1999;106:1262-1267.
2. Vryghem JC, Cleynenbreugel HV, Calster JV, Leroux K. Predicting cataract surgery results using a macular function test. *J Cataract Refract Surg*. 2004;30:2349-2353.
3. Chang MA, Airiani S, Miele D, Braunstein RE. A comparison of the potential acuity meter (PAM) and the illuminated near card (INC) in patients undergoing phacoemulsification. *Eye*. 2006;20(12):1345-1351. Epub 2005 Sep 23.

QUESTION 2

WHEN CAN CATARACT SURGERY ALONE BE PERFORMED IN PATIENTS WITH FUCHS' DYSTROPHY?

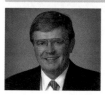

Walter J. Stark, MD

Fuchs' corneal dystrophy[1] (Figure 2-1) is a dominantly inherited, progressive disorder that affects the corneal endothelium. It is usually first observed in patients older than 50 years of age but can be seen in some patients in childhood. There is a progressive loss of endothelial cells with a secretion of an abnormally thickened basement membrane, leading to guttata formation. These guttata are often best seen by retroillumination but can be seen by direct illumination of the slit lamp.

Cataract surgery in patients with Fuchs' corneal dystrophy presents a challenge because the intraocular surgery can result in an 8% to 10% loss of the endothelial cells. The use of dispersive viscoelastics may lessen endothelial cell loss during surgery.

The decision as to whether to perform cataract surgery alone or cataract surgery plus penetrating keratoplasty (PK) or Descemet stripping automated endothelial keratoplasty (DSAEK) is often complex and depends on the assessment of endothelial cell health. It is debated whether the best assessment is by endothelial cell counts or central corneal pachymetry. In our practice, we have found that endothelial cell counts vary significantly and are not helpful in determining when a cornea with Fuchs' endothelial dystrophy might decompensate with cataract surgery. Therefore, we rely on clinical appearance of the cornea (epithelial edema versus no edema), the pachymetry measurements of the cornea, and the visual needs of the patient.

Past publications, including the American Academy of Ophthalmology's Preferred Practice Pattern[2] and the Basic and Clinical Science manual[3] for ophthalmologists, have indicated that a preoperative corneal thickness of >0.60 mm (600 μm) may be predictive of corneal decompensation and indicates that an initial PK may be required in these patients

Figure 2-1. An eye with Fuchs' corneal dystrophy.

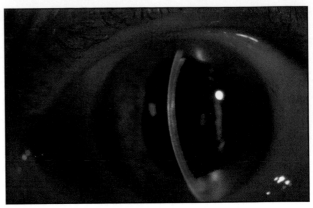

in combination with cataract surgery. Our experience at the Wilmer Eye Institute indicates that many patients with a preoperative corneal thickness of >600 µm, as measured by pachymetry, do very well after cataract surgery and do not require postoperative PK.

We recently published a 12-year review of 136 patients with Fuchs' dystrophy who underwent phacoemulsification and intraocular lens implantation.[4] The average preoperative corneal thickness in these patients was 580 µm, and 50 eyes (36.8%) had preoperative corneal thickness >600 µm. Postoperatively, the average visual acuity of our patients was 20/33. None of the eyes with a preoperative corneal thickness of <600 µm decompensated within 2 years after cataract surgery. Of the 50 patients with preoperative pachymetry measurements >600 µm, only 5 (10%) progressed to PK and 90% of the 50 eyes did not need a corneal transplant at least within the first 1 year to 2 years after cataract surgery. These patients had an average visual acuity of 20/35 postoperatively.

Based on these results, we suggest that the Preferred Practice Pattern for ophthalmologists extend the indications for cataract surgery in patients with Fuchs' dystrophy without obvious epithelial edema to undergoing cataract extraction without keratoplasty if the corneal thickness is <640 µm. Patients should be counseled that they have an approximately 10% chance of needing a keratoplasty within the first 1 year to 2 years after surgery and if they live long enough, they may eventually need a PK or DSAEK because this is a progressive disorder.

We modify our viscoelastic use during surgery in patients with Fuchs' dystrophy and use a dispersive viscoelastic such as Viscoat (Alcon, Inc, Fort Worth, Tex) or Healon 5 (Advanced Medical Optics, Santa Ana, Calif), which offer better protection of the endothelium during the phacoemulsification portion of the surgery. No study has been performed to definitively show that this is beneficial, but it is our belief that a dispersive viscoelastic helps protect the endothelium. One disadvantage of the dispersive viscoelastic is that it may trap small nuclear fragments in the peripheral angle that are not removed during phacoemulsification and/or irrigation-aspiration of the remaining viscoelastic. The retention of small nuclear fragments in the anterior chamber angle after cataract surgery can be damaging to the endothelium and can cause decompensation of the cornea. Therefore, the surgeon must be very careful to remove all nuclear chips during the cataract extraction and/or irrigation-aspiration.

In the past, we have performed cataract extraction alone in patients with Fuchs' dystrophy and a central corneal thickness of <640 µm. We realize that an increase in corneal thickness does lead to an increase in light scatter. We have found in our studies that visual acuity begins to deteriorate as the corneal thickness goes above 640 µm. We also reported on 12 patients who had a corneal thickness between 640 µm to 680 µm and underwent very careful cataract surgery. These were elderly and/or one-eyed patients in whom we thought PK was not warranted. Ten of the 12 cases (86%) maintained clear corneas at 2 years after surgery, with a median visual acuity of 20/40. There seems to be a correlation of increased corneal thickness of over 640 µm with a decrease in visual acuity, and currently we are evaluating this in a large number of Fuchs' dystrophy patients after cataract surgery.

Even with a relatively normal corneal thickness, if a patient has epithelial edema, then the cornea has decompensated and a PK or DSAEK is indicated. The surgeon can determine epithelial edema by retroillumination view and/or by applying a cotton-tipped applicator to the corneal epithelium after using anesthesia to see if it is detached, indicating epithelial edema.

The recent development and popularization of DSAEK by Melles,[5] Terry,[6-9] and Price[10] will certainly decrease the number of PKs for Fuchs' corneal dystrophy. Despite the success of DSAEK, we still recommend a simple cataract operation if there is no epithelial edema and central corneal thickness is <640 µm. In many of our patients, this has provided 20/20 visual acuity with a 90% chance of not needing a corneal transplant. If there is epithelial edema and the corneal thickness rises above 640 µm, there will be decreased visual acuity due to light scatter from the stroma and epithelial edema. In these cases, we now recommend a combination of phacoemulsification removal of the cataract and DSAEK. If the case is borderline or if the patient has one eye and cataract surgery might provide an improvement but possibly not a perfect visual acuity due to mild corneal edema, then we suggest cataract extraction alone to see what visual acuity is obtained. If it is adequate for the patient's needs, a PK or DSAEK can be avoided. If visual acuity is not adequate, then the patient can be treated with DSAEK. Although DSAEK is becoming more popular, there are complications of the procedure. A recent eye bank presentation in Toronto, Canada, June 2005 indicated that possibly 20% of DSAEKs dislocate. Our percentage of dislocation is less than 10%. Terry has recently reported a < 2% dislocation rate in the last 200 cases (personal communication, January 2007) and Price, a 14% dislocation rate[10] that has recently dropped to <1%. We have seen 2 cases in 40 present with rejection and both of these have cleared.

Conclusion

We have extended the indications for cataract surgery without simultaneous corneal surgery in eyes without epithelial edema to a corneal thickness of <640 µm and possibly to 680 µm. The ability to perform DSAEK, which is less debilitating to the patient than PK, has encouraged us to extend the indications for cataract extraction in patients with moderate Fuchs' dystrophy but without epithelial edema, realizing that DSAEK can be performed later if the patient does not achieve adequate visual acuity with cataract surgery alone.

References

1. Vogt A. Weitere Ergebnisse der spaltlampenmikroskopie des vorden bulbusabschnittes. *Albrecht Von Graefes Arch Klin Exp Ophthalmol.* 1921;106:63-103.
2. American Academy of Ophthalmology Anterior Segment Panel. Preferred practice pattern. Cataract in the adult eye. San Francisco: American Academy of Ophthalmology; 2001. Available at: http//www.aao.org/aao/education/library/ppp/index. cfm. Accessed October 1, 2002.
3. Basic and Clinical Science Course Section 11. Lens and cataract. San Francisco: American Academy of Ophthalmology; 2001.
4. Seitzman GD, Gottsch, JD, Stark WJ. Cataract surgery in patients with Fuchs' corneal dystrophy. *Ophthalmology.* 2005;112:441-446.
5. Melles GR, Wijdh RH, Nieuwendaal CP. A technique to excise the Descemet membrane from a recipient cornea (descemetorhexis). *Cornea.* 2004;23(3):286-288.
6. Terry MA, Ousley PJ. Corneal endothelial transplantation: advances in the surgical management of endothelial dysfunction. *Contemporary Ophthalmology.* 2002;1:1-8.
7. Ousley PJ, Terry MA. Stability of vision, topography, and endothelial density from 1 to 2 years after deep lamellar endothelial keratoplasty. *Ophthalmology.* 2005;112:50-57.
8. Terry MA. Endothelial keratoplasty: history, current state, and future directions. Cornea. 2006;25(8):873-878.
9. Terry MA. Management of Corneal Endothelial Dysfunction. AAO Specialty Clinical Update. Available at: http://www.aao.org/vp/edu/ced_cornea/v1m5. Accessed October 1, 2002.
10. Price FW, Price MO. Descemet's stripping with endothelial keratoplasty in 200 eyes: early challenges and technique to enhance donor adherence. *J Cataract Refract Surg.* 2006;32:411-418.

WHAT SHOULD I DO DIFFERENTLY FOR GLAUCOMA PATIENTS?

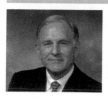

Bradford J. Shingleton, MD

As the general population ages, all ophthalmologists must be increasingly prepared to simultaneously manage cataract and glaucoma. Certain management issues are unique to either cataract or glaucoma individually and others share common concerns.

Preoperative Considerations

A cataract's impact on visual acuity can occasionally be difficult to assess in the setting of a miotic pupil or a glaucoma patient with significant optic nerve damage. Maximal dilation, potential acuity testing, and brightness acuity testing all help to facilitate such assessment.

The type of glaucoma and degree of optic nerve damage can also be difficult to assess because the cataract can obscure the view of the optic nerve and compromise visual field testing. Be sure to get the most objective analysis of optic nerve damage as possible prior to cataract surgery because this will help determine the choice of operation and therapeutic adjuncts that might be employed intraoperatively and postoperatively.

The impact of cataract surgery on intraocular pressure (IOP) in eyes with glaucoma is important to consider preoperatively. Temporal small incision phacoemulsification procedures have a statistically significant, but small, IOP-lowering effect in normal eyes, glaucoma suspect eyes, and glaucoma eyes.[1] Trabeculectomy, when performed first, increases the risk of subsequent cataract formation. This is particularly the case when there is a shallow chamber or significant inflammation postoperatively. Subsequent cataract surgery performed in the setting of prior trabeculectomy tends to raise the IOP a modest amount in these eyes.[2] Traditional thinking suggests that surgical intervention for glaucoma may be less effective in the pseudophakic eye than in the phakic eye. This may be true in eyes with scarred conjunctiva compared to those eyes with normal conjunctiva, but satisfactory IOP control can be achieved with filtration surgery in pseudophakic eyes that have mobile conjunctiva.[3] All these points must be taken into account when determining the initial procedure of choice for coexisting cataract and glaucoma. Combined cataract and glaucoma procedures remain an option for all eyes.

Traditional dogma has taught that argon laser trabeculoplasty (ALT) and most likely selective laser trabeculoplasty (SLT) are more effective in phakic eyes than pseudophakic eyes. Indeed, there is a statistically significant greater reduction in IOP after ALT in phakic eyes compared to pseudophakic eyes. However, there is not a substantial clinical difference. ALT may still be used after cataract surgery with the anticipation that IOP reduction can still be clinically significant.[4] ALT and SLT do not blunt early postoperative IOP elevation that may occur after cataract surgery, and cataract surgery itself does not appear to diminish the IOP-lowering effect of ALT if performed after laser treatment. In short, the indications for ALT or SLT in the glaucoma patient with a cataract are basically the same as for any glaucoma patient.

If you decide to perform cataract surgery alone or a combined cataract and glaucoma procedure, it is appropriate to provide antibiotic prophylaxis for at least 3 days preoperatively. I favor the newest generation fluoroquinolones. I also supplement with topical nonsteroidal anti-inflammatory drops for the same period of time. If patients are on miotics, it is helpful to stop them at least 1 week preoperatively and to add a nonsteroidal anti-inflammatory agent with the usual dilation program on the day of surgery, particularly if iris manipulation is anticipated. Topical prostaglandin agents generally do not have to be stopped prior to cataract surgery. However, if the eye is injected or inflamed, as can occasionally occur with topical prostaglandin agents or other glaucoma medicines, it may be helpful to stop the offending drops to reduce external conjunctival inflammation. This is particularly important if a simultaneous cataract and glaucoma procedure is to be performed. Any glaucoma procedure that depends on conjunctival filtration will potentially be compromised in the setting of conjunctival inflammation. Benzalkonium chloride and other preservatives can also be toxic to the conjunctiva and this must be kept in mind when preparing glaucoma eyes for cataract surgery. Cessation of anticoagulation medicines such as warfarin may be considered with combined cataract and glaucoma surgery but is rarely required for cataract surgery alone. If significant ocular inflammation is present preoperatively, topical steroids may be helpful prior to surgery. Systemic steroids may be indicated for significantly inflamed eyes.

Intraoperative Considerations

The surgical site for cataract surgery in the setting of glaucoma is best placed temporally. This avoids conjunctival manipulation superiorly in case future filtration surgery is required. Either clear-cornea or scleral tunnel incisions from the temporal aspect are both associated with IOP reduction postoperatively and do not compromise subsequent filtration surgery as long as the superior conjunctiva is not violated.

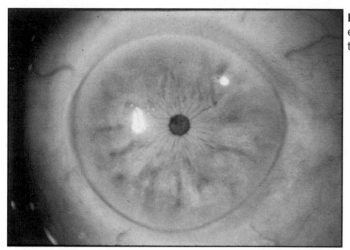

Figure 3-1. Miotic pupil requiring enlargement for phacoemulsification.

The miotic pupil (Figure 3-1) is a common finding in glaucoma patients. I see this most commonly in patients who have been on chronic miotics and in pseudoexfoliation patients. The intraoperative floppy iris syndrome (IFIS) has been well described and details for IFIS management are dealt with in Question 25.

The goal in managing the miotic pupil is to achieve adequate surgical pupil size while still maintaining near normal pupillary reactivity and contour postoperatively. Intraoperative techniques for management of the miotic pupil start with epinephrine in the infusion bottle. Peripupillary membranes should be stripped prior to releasing synechiae. These veneer-like membranes are occasionally present in patients who have been on long-term miotics. Posterior synechiae should then be swept and released. Viscoelastic expansion of the pupil after sweeping and releasing synechiae is often sufficient to achieve satisfactory pupillary size.

Bimanual pupil stretching without sphincterotomies is a simple and safe technique for enlarging the pupil. In my hands, this achieves a satisfactory result in over 90% of cases. I do not recommend iris stretching in patients at risk for IFIS. When performing bimanual iris stretching, a slow, steady bimanual stretch to the limbal area is recommended in the 12:00 to 6:00 and 9:00 to 3:00 meridians (Figure 3-2). This is a microsphincterotomy technique that results in excellent preservation of pupillary function and contour. Mechanical Beehler-style pupillary dilating instruments with either 4-point or 2-point fixation can be used with the same net effect. Self-retaining pupil expansion rings are highly effective and probably achieve the greatest pupillary expansion. They take a little more time intraoperatively to place and are not suited for reuse.

Self-retaining iris retractors (titanium or flexible nylon) are highly effective and can be easily placed via paracentesis incisions. Sequential, gradual retraction of the hook retractors minimizes sphincter tears. The resultant shape created by the hooks can be either a diamond or rectangle (relative to the wound) depending on the zone where pupillary expansion is most needed. When using the rectangle configuration, relaxing the proximal hooks prior to phacoemulsification may decrease iris contact with the phacoemulsifier. Scissors sphincterotomies, sphincterectomies, and sector iridectomies may be indicated in selected circumstances.

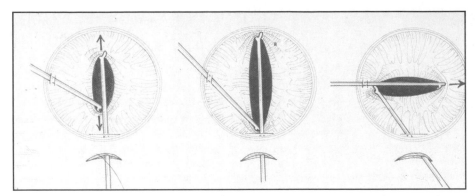

Figure 3-2. Bimanual pupil stretch. (Reprinted with permission from Masket S, Crandall A. *Atlas of Cataract Surgery.* Oxford, United Kingdom: Informa Healthcare; 1999.)

Pseudoexfoliation warrants special attention since this is so common in glaucoma patients. In our studies involving a large number of pseudoexfoliation patients, the incidence of zonule dehiscence approaches 2.5% in pseudoexfoliation syndrome and is much lower in nonpseudoexfoliation eyes.[5] Preoperative clues to zonule problems include phacodonesis, anterior chamber depth asymmetry, visibility of the lens equator on eccentric gaze, decentered nucleus on primary gaze, iridolenticular gap, and a very shallow chamber. Intraoperative clues include a "pseudoelastic capsule" that is resistant to capsule puncture and radiating capsule striae that extend to the periphery during capsulorrhexis. Anterior chamber depth instability and dramatic anterior-posterior displacement of the lens are also important signs.

Intraoperative surgical techniques that might be considered in high-risk pseudoexfoliation eyes include a posterior limbal or scleral tunnel incision if there is a greater likelihood of zonular instability or for the need to enlarge the incision for a backup intraocular lens (IOL). Effective hydrodissection and hydrolineation reduce the need to direct the phaco tip near the capsular fornix where the lax capsule and zonules are prone to aspiration. Phacoemulsification maneuvers should minimize any downward pressure on the nucleus. Capsule tension rings and capsule tension segments may be very helpful. It is important to appreciate, however, that nonsutured capsule tension rings can still be associated with late IOL decentration, subluxation, or even dislocation. Postoperative anterior capsule contraction should be treated with neodymium:yttrium-aluminum-garnet laser anterior capsulotomy to reduce the chance of IOL displacement.

Postoperative Considerations

Postoperative IOP is obviously important to monitor in all patients with glaucoma. The time period from 2 hours to 8 hours postoperatively may hold the greatest risk for an IOP spike. If there is particular concern for IOP elevation in glaucoma patients, intracameral carbachol may be the most effective pharmacological adjunct for blunting postoperative IOP rise. The use of a topical beta-blocker, alpha agonist, and/or miotic at the conclusion of surgery and topical/systemic carbonic anhydrase inhibitors may also be indicated. It is questionable whether prostaglandin agents at the time of surgery have a significant impact on postoperative IOP elevation. If possible, it is best to avoid periocular injection of long-acting steroids because of the possibility of a steroid response following surgery. Steroid response usually develops several weeks postoperatively, but occasionally can present earlier and should be kept in mind if IOP elevations occur in the early-to-mid postoperative period. For significant IOP elevations that occur on the first postoperative day, sterile release of aqueous via a paracentesis incision (with preoperative administration of topical antibiotics and povidone) can significantly reduce IOP. However, the effect may be transient and IOP should be monitored in the office after release of aqueous via the paracentesis site.[6]

In glaucoma patients having cataract surgery alone, I favor stopping all glaucoma medications postoperatively if the IOP is satisfactory on the first postoperative visit. Resumption of glaucoma medicines is based on IOP, optic nerve configuration, and visual field loss. If medications are required, I favor adding medicines in the following order: topical aqueous suppressants, alpha agonists, prostaglandin agonists, and miotics. Prostaglandin agonists are unlikely to cause cystoid macular edema if the cataract surgery has been uncomplicated, but it may be appropriate to delay their administration in the early postoperative phase for this reason.

In uncomplicated cataract surgery in normal, glaucoma suspect, and glaucoma patients, a 1 mm to 3 mm decrease in IOP can be anticipated for up to 5 years postoperatively. IOP in glaucoma patients tends to rise back to pretreatment levels by 5 years postoperatively, but medication requirements may still be reduced. There is no question that the beneficial effect of phacoemulsification on IOP has changed our criteria for decision making in patients with cataract and glaucoma. Combined cataract and glaucoma surgery may still be indicated and filtration surgery prior to cataract surgery may be appropriate in highly compromised eyes, such as those with active inflammation or neovascular glaucoma. However, phacoemulsification alone is often a highly satisfactory procedure in terms of visual rehabilitation and IOP control.

References

1. Shingleton BJ, Gamell LS, O'Donoghue MW, Baylus SL, King R. Long-term changes in intraocular pressure after clear-corneal phacoemulsification. Normal patients versus glaucoma suspect and glaucoma patients. *J Cataract Refract Surg.* 1999;24:885-890.
2. Shingleton BJ, O'Donoghue MW, Hall PE. Results of phacoemulsification in eyes with pre-existing glaucoma filters. *J Cataract Refract Surg.* 2003;29:1093-1096.
3. Shingleton BJ, Alfano C, O'Donoghue MW, Rivera J. Efficacy of glaucoma filtration surgery in pseudophakic patients with or without conjunctival scarring. *J Cataract Refract Surg.* 2004;30:2504-2509.
4. Shingleton BJ, Richter CU, Dharma S, et al. Long term efficacy of argon laser trabeculoplasty—10-year follow-up. *Ophthalmology.* 1993;100:1324-1329.
5. Shingleton BJ, Heltzer J, O'Donoghue MW. Outcomes of phacoemulsification in patients with and without pseudoexfoliation syndrome. *J Cataract Refract Surg.* 2003;29:1080-1086.
6. Hildebrand GD, Wickremasinghe SS, Tranus PG, Harris ML, Little BC. Efficacy of anterior chamber decompression in controlling early intraocular pressure spikes after uneventful phacoemulsification. *J Cataract Refract Surg.* 2003;29:1087-1092.

WHICH PATIENTS NEED A COMBINED GLAUCOMA PROCEDURE?

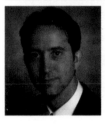

Thomas Samuelson, MD

The presentation of coincident cataract and glaucoma is one of the most common clinical challenges facing the anterior segment surgeon. While the only effective therapeutic intervention for cataract is surgical, glaucoma may be effectively managed either medically or surgically. As such, when you make the decision to surgically intervene for cataract in a patient with glaucoma, you must also determine whether to continue medical management of the glaucoma or perform combined cataract and glaucoma surgery.

Recent advances in the medical management of glaucoma have significantly reduced the number of combined glaucoma procedures that are performed (Figure 4-1). Better glaucoma medications have led to an increase in the percentage of patients that may be managed with cataract surgery alone. Indeed, it is well known that cataract surgery alone lowers intraocular pressure (IOP), at least transiently, in a significant percentage of cases.[1]

Nevertheless, the glaucoma-combined procedure remains an extremely important option for some patients. While there are exceptions, I prefer coincident cataract and glaucoma surgery in the following situations:

* Visually significant cataract and…

    ❖ glaucoma that is poorly controlled despite medical therapy.

    ❖ progressive glaucoma in patients that are noncompliant or cannot afford medications.

    ❖ progressive glaucoma in patients that are intolerant of medications.

    ❖ stable or progressive glaucoma in patients on 3 or more glaucoma medications.

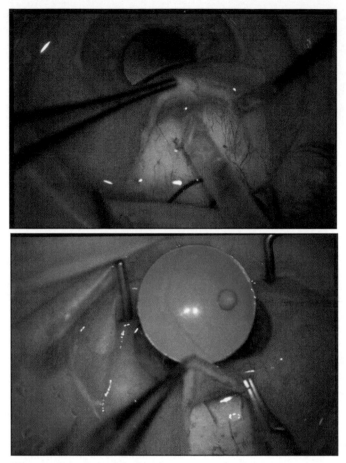

Figure 4-1. Coincident cataract and glaucoma surgery remains an important option for patients with both cataract and glaucoma. Both procedures may be performed via one site (shown here) or with separate incisions.

❖ stable, medically controlled glaucoma in a patient who chooses to reduce or eliminate the need for glaucoma medications.

In such cases, the cataract is the primary indication for surgery (ie, an individual with glaucoma has a visually significant cataract requiring surgery). The surgeon must then decide how to manage the glaucoma. However, there are also situations in which glaucoma surgery is indicated and the surgeon must decide how to manage the lens. This decision is clear-cut in many instances. For example, the presence of a significant cataract in the setting of a planned glaucoma surgery is an indication for combined surgery. In general, my indications for lens removal are more liberal in patients scheduled for planned glaucoma surgery. For example, I will remove a marginally significant cataract during a planned trabeculectomy, knowing that the cataract will likely progress following the glaucoma surgery.

Once the decision is made to proceed with combined cataract and glaucoma surgery, several management decisions must be made. While phacoemulsification is the cataract procedure of choice, there are several options for the surgical management of glaucoma. Each of these procedures can be combined with phacoemulsification as part of a glaucoma-combined procedure.

Trabeculectomy

Coincident phacoemulsification and trabeculectomy remains the gold standard of combined glaucoma procedures. Modern small incision cataract surgery is an ideal adjunct to trabeculectomy. Some surgeons prefer single incision surgery, while others favor separate sites for the trabeculectomy and cataract procedure. Most published studies suggest that single-site or 2-site surgery is equally efficacious.[2] I regularly use both strategies depending on the clinical situation. For example, in eyes with excellent surgical exposure and well-dilated pupils, I usually prefer single-site surgery. Single-site surgery is efficient and efficacious and obviates the need for a corneal suture. Two-site surgery is indicated when surgical exposure is suboptimal or when the surgeon simply feels less comfortable performing cataract surgery from a superior approach. I also prefer 2-site surgery when the pupil fails to dilate well. Typically, these are patients on systemic alpha-1 blockers such as tamsulosin (Flomax, Boehringer Ingelheim Pharmaceuticals, Inc, Ridgefield, Conn), who have pseudoexfoliation syndrome, or have bound down pupils. In these cases, a clear corneal incision provides a more anterior entry into the anterior chamber and the iris is less likely to prolapse into the wound. When clear corneal surgery is performed in the setting of trabeculectomy, I strongly favor placing a suture in the corneal wound due to the fact that one cannot be certain that the early postoperative IOP will be sufficient to adequately seal the corneal incision.

The Search for a New Procedure

While early to midterm postoperative results of trabeculectomy are excellent, bleb survival remains vulnerable to the healing whims of the conjunctiva, often resulting in late failures. Conjunctiva in its natural state is prone to scarring, contraction, and ultimately bleb failure. While antimetabolites such as mitomycin C and 5-fluorouracil greatly enhance the success of trabeculectomy, the avascular or thinned conjunctiva is more prone to late bleb leaks, hypotony, and—perhaps most concerning—late bleb infection.

Blebless Glaucoma Surgery

A surgical procedure that lowers IOP without requiring a filtration bleb would be highly desirable. Such a procedure would eliminate much of the risk and morbidity inherent to traditional bleb-based, transscleral filtration procedures. Viscocanalostomy and nonpenetrating deep sclerectomy (NPDS) were conceived with this goal in mind. Stegmann lead a resurgence of interest in viscocanalostomy in the late 1990s.[3] While the Stegmann viscocanalostomy is truly "blebless," most versions of NPDS still create a filtration bleb. Both procedures rely on the flow of aqueous through an exquisitely thin "trabeculo-Descemet" membrane. Such procedures are technically difficult to perform and, like trabeculectomy, may be prone to late scarring. Accordingly, they have not been widely adopted. Nether the less, nonpenetrating surgery is an acceptably safe and effective procedure to lower IOP and can be combined with phacoemulsification. Perhaps more importantly, with the renewed interest in procedures involving Schlemm's canal, these procedures have paved the way for newer and more technologically sophisticated devices that bypass the trabecular meshwork (TM) and facilitate flow of aqueous directly into the canal itself.

Trabecular Bypass Devices

Trabecular bypass stents and shunts are investigational devices that represent the most recent efforts toward achieving blebless glaucoma surgery. Such procedures are based on the premise that the pathology in the physiological outflow system is in the juxtacanalicular portion of the meshwork or within the inner wall itself. By bypassing the proximal TM, these procedures facilitate flow of aqueous into Schlemm's canal by shunting (GMP EyePass, GMP Surgical Solutions, Fort Lauderdale, Fla) or stenting (Glaukos iStent, Glaukos Corp, Laguna Hills, Calif) the canal itself. Other devices such as the Solx Gold Shunt (Solx Inc, Boston, Mass) divert aqueous into the suprachoroidal space. Excimer laser trabeculostomy (ELT) utilizes the excimer laser to ablate trabecular tissue and provide a direct communication of aqueous into Schlemm's canal. While currently investigational, such procedures can be performed coincident to cataract surgery as part of a glaucoma-combined procedure and may play an increasingly important role in this setting.

Potential Pitfalls

While the concept of trabecular bypass is intriguing and indeed promising, much work remains to be done. Some investigators have expressed concern over the lack of circumferential flow within Schlemm's canal. In other words, even if the TM is successfully bypassed with a stent or shunt, there is evidence to suggest that the outflow enhancement may be limited to several clock-hours surrounding the stent or perhaps a single quadrant. In this case, multiple stents or shunts may be needed to adequately lower IOP. Alternatively, the circumferential flow may be enhanced by microcannulation of the canal by newly developed, investigational techniques such as the iScience 360-degree viscocanulation (iScience Interventional, Menlo Park, Calif).

Endoscopic Cyclophotocoagulation

Endoscopic cyclophotocoagulation (ECP) is yet another option for the coincident management of cataract and glaucoma. The procedure is performed through a clear corneal incision and is tailor made as an adjunct to cataract surgery because access to the ciliary processes is greatly enhanced in pseudophakic eyes. Despite the lack of any prospective randomized trials, this technique has become popular for the management of milder forms of glaucoma to reduce the burden of medical therapy. While I prefer to lower IOP by enhancing outflow, there may be a role for ECP in the reduction of IOP in select patients.

Conclusion

The simultaneous presentation of cataract and glaucoma remains one of the most common comorbidities facing the anterior segment surgeon. The surgical options continue to evolve and improve. The management decisions should be individualized to both the patient and the surgeon to maximize outcomes and minimize risk. Ultimately, we are in a period of transition, and change may be the only constant as our medical and surgical options continue to improve.

References

1. Mathalone N, Hyamus M, Neiman S, Buckman G, Hod Y, Geyer O. Long-term intraocular pressure control after clear corneal phacoemulsification in glaucoma patients. *J Cataract Refract Surg.* 2005;31(3):479-483.
2. Shingleton BJ, Price RS, O'Donoghue MW, Goyal S. Comparison of 1-site versus 2-site phacotrabeculectomy. *J Cataract Refract Surg.* 2006;32(5):799-802.
3. Stegmann R, Pienaar A, Miller D. Viscocanalostomy for open-angle glaucoma in black African patients. *J Cataract Refractive Surg.* 1999;25:316-322.
4. Shaarawy T, Mansouri K, Schnyder C, Ravinet E, Achache F, Mermoud A. Long-term results of deep sclerectomy with collagen implant. *J Cataract Refract Surg.* 2004;30(6):1225-1231.

WHAT SHOULD I DO DIFFERENTLY IN PATIENTS AT HIGHER RISK FOR RETINAL DETACHMENT?

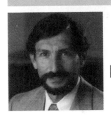

Richard J. Mackool, MD

Retrospective studies indicate that males with an axial length of 25.0 mm or more have the greatest risk for retinal detachment (RD) after cataract removal. Although the reported rate varies, data from my practice indicate that a male between 20 and 60 years of age with an axial length of 25.0 mm or greater has an RD risk of approximately 4.8% during the first 3 years after cataract-implant surgery. Women with axial myopia have a much lower risk of RD. My data indicate that women with an axial length of 25.0 mm or greater and between 20 and 60 years of age have approximately a 0.3% risk of RD during the first 3 years after cataract removal (Figure 5-1).

The risk for RD is almost certainly less if a posterior vitreous detachment (PVD) is already present. Because older patients are more likely to have had a PVD, their risk of RD is significantly decreased. Interestingly, the RD rate, in our data, remained approximately the same regardless of axial length beyond 25.0 mm. Most RDs occurred within the first year after cataract-implant surgery and very few developed during the first 2 months.

There is no evidence of varying risk of RD with IOL type or design, nor is there evidence of increased risk after YAG laser capsulotomy if the intraocular lens (IOL) has been placed within the capsular sac (independent studies performed by Howard Gimbel, MD[1] and Richard Mackool, MD). Because some patients who develop RD may require intraocular silicone oil, it is probably best to use an acrylic or polymethylmethacrylate (PMMA) IOL in patients more likely to develop RD to avoid the potential problem of silicone oil deposition on the posterior IOL surface in these eyes.

Peer-reviewed literature indicates that only patients with a symptomatic flap tear of the retina require treatment and that treatment of either an asymptomatic tear or a

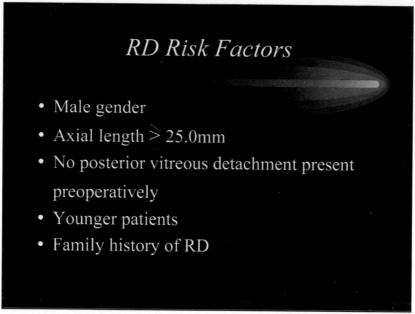

Figure 5-1. RD risk factors.

symptomatic nonflap tear does not reduce the risk of subsequent RD.[2] Therefore, asymptomatic patients would not be expected to benefit from either preoperative or postoperative retinal consultation. Unfortunately, this appears to be of greater medicolegal importance than a matter of appropriate medical practice.

There is no evidence that the type of phacoemulsification procedure performed (ie, coaxial versus microcoaxial, bimanual microincisional cataract surgery) has any effect on the incidence of RD. Conjecture that certain procedures result in less posterior capsule "trampolining" is at best anecdotal and clearly unproven. Furthermore, the delayed nature of RD after uneventful phacoemulsification procedures would appear to argue against such an intraoperative mechanism as a factor.

If the vitreous cavity contains silicone oil at the time of phacoemulsification, intraoperative anterior chamber shallowing may occur because of the buoyancy of the oil. This is of greatest concern after IOL insertion because loss of the anterior chamber could cause contact of the IOL with the corneal endothelium. This can be prevented by avoiding removal of viscoelastic from the anterior chamber with an irrigation/aspiration handpiece or even a bimanual technique. Rather, after IOL insertion, a small (25 gauge) chamber maintainer can be inserted through a puncture of approximately 0.5 mm, and the viscoelastic can be aspirated through a similar puncture, utilizing a syringe with a 27-gauge cannula. In this manner, the anterior chamber can be maintained as the viscoelastic is removed.

IOL implant power calculation in eyes containing silicone oil is complicated by difficulty obtaining accurate axial length measurements using ultrasonography. Optical coherence biometry (OCB) is much more accurate in these eyes. When silicone oil is present, the higher index of refraction of silicone will reduce the effective power of the posterior surface of an IOL. One option is to use an IOL with a posterior surface that has no power (ie, plano posterior surface). Otherwise, rather complex calculations must be made in order to derive the increased appropriate power for the IOL. If removal of the silicone oil is planned for a later date, it may be advisable to piggyback IOLs (one in the capsular sac and one in the sulcus). The latter implant can be removed at a later date, most likely at the time of silicone oil removal, in order to obtain the desired refractive effect as discussed below. The reader is referred to the American Academy of Ophthalmology publication *Focal Points*, Clinical Module Volume XXII, No. 9, September 2004 by Warren Hill, MD and Sandra Frazier Byrne for a thorough explanation and discussion of this subject.

Finally, because pseudophakia increases the risk of RD, all patients at greater risk should be counseled about this fact preoperatively, and it may be advisable to review the potential symptoms of a RD with the patient.

References

1. Van Westenbrugge JA, Gimbel HV, Souchek J, Chow D. Incidence of retinal detachment following DSAEK capsulotomy after cataract surgery. *J Cataract Refract Surg.* 1992;18(4):352-355.
2. Byer NE. The natural history of asymptomatic retinal breaks. *Ophthalmology.* 1982;89(9):1033-1039.

WITH HOW LARGE A ZONULAR DIALYSIS CAN PHACO BE PERFORMED?

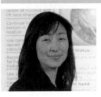

Bonnie An Henderson, MD

Surgery in the presence of a zonular dialysis can be a challenging situation for even the most experienced surgeon. The ability to perform small incision phacoemulsification with a zonular dialysis depends on the density of the lens and the stability and strength of the remaining zonules. If the patient is young and the lens is soft, the nucleus can most likely be removed with slow aspiration (Figure 6-1) even in the presence of a large dialysis if the remaining intact zonules are strong. Conversely, if the lens is brunescent in the setting of pseudoexfoliation (PXF), even a 2 clock-hour dialysis may be too large to complete successful phacoemulsification. The determination of whether to phacoemulsify the lens or to perform a large incision extraction is based on the combination of both preoperative and intraoperative findings (Table 6-1).

The first opportunity to diagnose zonular abnormalities is during the preoperative examination. A careful and thorough history should cover potential risk factors for zonular damage, such as trauma, previous ocular surgery, and systemic conditions such as Marfan's syndrome and homocystinuria. A history of prior vitrectomy and chronic silicone oil tamponade can also be associated with zonular weakness.[1]

At the slit-lamp examination, one should look carefully for PXF. Chamber shallowing despite a normal axial length may indicate zonular laxity in such patients. One method that I use to evaluate zonular integrity at the slit lamp is to have the person look in multiple directions and then straight ahead. If significant zonular weakness exists, one might see phacodonesis during these motility exercises. If phacodonesis is present, it can be assumed that at least 25% of the zonules are weakened. If the contralateral eye is pseudophakic, pseudophacodonesis may indicate the likelihood of zonular weakness in the

Figure 6-1. Traumatic cataract with zonular dialysis.

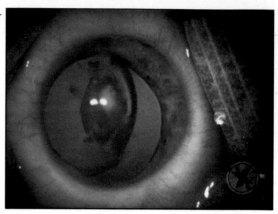

Table 6-1

Stepwise Approach to Evaluation of Zonular Dialysis

1. Careful history (trauma, silicone oil, systemic disease)
2. Preoperative evaluation (PXF, phacodonesis)
3. Patient consent/counseling
4. Preoperative planning—chondroitin sulfate, capsule staining, capsular hooks, capsular tension rings (CTRs), scleral tunnel, preoperative nonsteroidal anti-inflammatory drugs (NSAIDs)
5. Anesthesia considerations—peribulbar block rather than topical
6. Intraoperative evaluation—movement during capsulorrhexis, phaco
7. Intraoperative procedure—complete hydrodissection, hydrodelineation, supracapsular approach, use of chopper, placement of hooks, CTRs
8. Plan for conversion to extracapsular cataract extraction (ECCE)/intracapsular cataract extraction/pars plana vitrectomy (PPV), pars plana lensectomy (PPL)

preoperative eye. Finally, one should maximally dilate the pupil to visualize as much of the peripheral lens as possible.

If zonular weakness is suspected, proper informed consent is crucial in managing the patient's expectations. The patient must be made aware that both the surgery and the postoperative care may be more complicated and prolonged. The patient should also be counseled about the potential need for a vitrectomy, for dislocated lens fragments, and for the greater risk of retinal detachment and cystoid macular edema with vitreous loss. I will often paint the worst-case scenario for patients so they will expect the worst and hopefully be pleasantly surprised.

In cases of zonular dialysis, preoperative planning becomes even more important. In these patients, I will start topical NSAIDs for 1 week preoperatively because of the higher risk for intraoperative complications and postoperative cystoid macular edema. Anticipating a potentially longer operative time, I use peribulbar or retrobulbar anesthesia instead of topical anesthesia in these cases. This also makes it easier to convert to a manual ECCE if necessary.

In cases in which a large zonular dialysis is present, I will perform a scleral tunnel rather than a clear corneal incision to facilitate converting to a large-incision ECCE. The

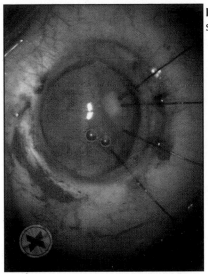

Figure 6-2. Photo of the same lens after placement of capsular hooks.

anterior capsule should be stained with either trypan blue or indocyanine green especially if capsular hooks are to be used. Of the various viscoelastics, chondroitin sulfate is best suited in cases with a zonular dialysis due to its dispersive/highly retentive properties. The chondroitin sulfate will push back the vitreous face and is not as quickly aspirated. The use of capsular hooks and CTRs will be discussed in a later chapter.

Intraoperative assessment of the degree of zonular dialysis begins when the eye is first manipulated. For example, phacodonesis might be noted during the conjunctival peritomy for preparation of the scleral tunnel incision. The degree of zonular integrity can also be evaluated during the capsulorrhexis. Puncturing the capsule with the cystotome and grasping the flap with the forceps often give the surgeon an accurate tactile sense of either normal or abnormal countertraction from the zonules. Any improper movement of the lens capsule during hydrodissection or lens sculpting should be noted. If a zonular dialysis is present, abundant chondroitin sulfate (dispersive) viscoelastic should be used to prevent anterior prolapse of the vitreous. Capsular hooks and CTRs can be placed before the start of phacoemulsification to stabilize the capsular bag and prevent vitreous prolapse (Figure 6-2).[2-4] The lens must be completely hydrodissected and hydrodelineated to decrease stress on the remaining zonules when the lens is manipulated. If the lens is not fully mobile within the capsular bag, a supracapsular phacotechnique should be considered. Avoid a 4-quadrant divide-and-conquer approach, which necessitates numerous rotations within the capsule. Instead, the use of phaco chopping methods is preferred in order to minimize stress on the zonules and capsular bag.

If the dialysis is greater than 3 clock hours, the lens is brunescent, the pupil dilates poorly, and the integrity of the remaining zonules is compromised, then phacoemulsification of the lens—even with the use of capsular hooks and CTRs—may not be the best approach. In these instances, it may be safer to remove the lens through a large incision manual extracapsular approach or even with a planned pars plana lensectomy-vitrectomy. When selecting a surgical approach in the presence of a zonular dialysis, one must consider other ocular variables such as pupil size, corneal endothelial health, lens density, and the surgeon's familiarity with using capsular hooks and CTRs.

References

1. Menapace R, Findl O, Georgopoulos M, Rainer G, Vass C, Schmetterer K. The capsular tension ring: designs, applications, and techniques. *J Cataract Refract Surg.* 2000;26:898-912.
2. Hara T, Hara T, Yamada Y. "Equator ring" for maintenance of the completely circular contour of the capsular bag equator after cataract removal. *Ophthalmic Surg.* 1991;22:358-359.
3. Legler UFC, Witschel BM. The capsular ring: a new device for complicated cataract surgery. Abstract F12. *Ger J Ophthalmol.* 1994;3:265.
4. Cionni RJ, Osher RH. Management of profound zonular dialysis or weakness with a new endocapsular ring designed for scleral fixation. *J Cataract Refract Surg.* 1998;24:1299-1306.

I HAVE A CATARACT PATIENT WITH A TRAUMATIC IRIS DEFECT AND GLARE SYMPTOMS. WHAT SHOULD I DO?

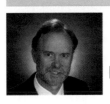

Francis W. Price, Jr, MD

Case management here depends on the type of iris defect and the extent of problems caused by the trauma. Suturing the defect partially or totally closed can treat many traumatic iris defects. Those not amenable to suturing can be treated with an artificial iris lens. Here are some basic things to check:

* Is the crystalline lens still well supported by the zonular apparatus? If less than one-third of the zonular apparatus is detached or weakened, then a capsular tension ring (CTR) (AMO, FCI, Morcher) can be implanted to stabilize the capsule during cataract surgery. If the crystalline lens is more unstable, consider implantation of a Cionni ring (Morcher, Stuttgart, Germany) along with a foldable IOL or complete removal of the lens with a pars plana vitrectomy-lensectomy and suture fixation of a CZ70BD lens (Alcon, Fort Worth, Tex) to the sclera.[1] Iris-fixated lenses can be used but may cause problems if the iris is already compromised.

* Is vitreous prolapse present? If so, at least some of the zonular fibers are absent. If the amount of vitreous prolapse is small, it may be possible to push the vitreous back with some combination of dense viscoelastic like Healon V (Advanced Medical Optics, Santa Ana, Calif) and a dispersive viscoelastic like Viscoat (Alcon, Fort Worth, Tex). If the amount of vitreous prolapse is substantial, a vitrectomy may be necessary. I prefer a pars plana vitrectomy because it permits the use of a fiberoptic light source without distorting the cornea. Compared with an anterior approach, the pars plana approach allows more complete removal of the vitreous so as to better avoid postoperative vitreous strands to the corneal/scleral phaco incision.

❋ What is the status of the iris and the defect? This influences the choice of implant and incision size.

❋ Careful evaluation of the iris consistency is essential. Does the iris have a normal consistency? An iris that is fibrotic or one that is friable and wispy is not a good candidate for suturing. The former will not respond to manipulation and sutures will pull through the latter, leaving ragged remnants. Irides can still be in good shape years after an injury, but examine them closely.

❋ Is the pupillary sphincter still functional?

❋ Are there peripheral anterior synechiae (PAS) or posterior synechiae (PS) that need to be lysed?

❋ Is there an iridodialysis? If so, how many clock hours?

❋ Is any iris tissue missing from an earlier surgery (eg, was any removed after prolapse out of the eye)?

We will now discuss how to handle these problems. Every case of traumatic cataract with iris abnormalities is different, so these will be general guidelines.

In cases with missing iris tissue, evaluate the consistency of the iris as described above. If it can hold sutures, it can be closed with polypropylene sutures. However, very large defects can be difficult to close even with normal iris tissue consistency. Intraoperative problems can be caused by suturing a defect closed in a soft underinflated eye. As the eye is reinflated, the sutures might cheesewire through the tissue or might cause an iris dialysis with bleeding. In soft eyes, one must allow enough room for expansion of the iris when the eye is inflated. Iris defects should be sutured after cataract removal and IOL placement because the closure will likely make the iris tenser and the pupil smaller. Iris suturing can be done within a closed eye to avoid problems like re-expansion of the eye pulling on the sutures. Passing sutures either on curved or straight needles can be done with a technique similar to that of placing McCannell sutures.

What if little or no iris is present or the iris that is present is fibrotic or friable? If it looks like the iris defect cannot be repaired with sutures, then one can use an artificial iris implant to block the defect that is causing the symptoms (Figure 7-1). Currently, the only type I use is the Model 311 lens (Ophtec, Groningen, The Netherlands). It is the only artificial iris implant undergoing a Food and Drug Administration (FDA) study to obtain marketing approval for general use,[2] and we hope it will gain approval in the next few years. Morcher makes a number of designs, all black, and to my knowledge none are involved in FDA studies. This means that these are only available with an FDA compassionate use exemption and Institutional Review Board approval.

The Model 311 artificial iris implant comes in 3 colors (blue, green, and brown) and has a 4-mm central optic, which is available plano or in powers ranging from +10 D to 30 D. This 9-mm diameter polymethylmethacrylate (PMMA) implant requires a 10-mm incision. The haptics are 13.75 mm in overall diameter so that they can be placed in the sulcus if good support is present. If not, the haptics also have eyelets to allow suture fixation to the sclera. The Model 311 IOL can be placed in the capsular bag but this is not for the faint-of-heart because it requires good zonular support with about a 6.5-mm capsulotomy (see Figure 7-1).

Placing the Model 311 artificial iris lens in either the bag or sulcus is straightforward. However, in cases in which it needs to be suture fixated to the sclera,[1] there are some

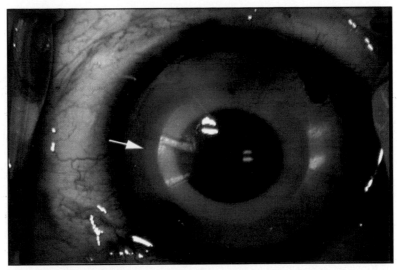

Figure 7-1. Implantation of an Ophtec Model 311 artificial iris lens in the capsular bag for treatment of cataract and complete iris loss. This patient suffered a traumatic injury, which broke open prior radial keratotomy incisions and caused iris extrusion, lens opacification, and zonular damage. After CTR placement and phacoemulsification, a Model 311 lens was implanted in the capsular bag. The capsular bag was stained with trypan blue ophthalmic solution to improve visualization; an arrow indicates the edge of the capsulorrhexis. With placement in the bag, the haptics curled down over the edge of the implant.

important tips. First, use 9-0 polypropylene, not 10-0. The ciliary body degrades the suture.[3] 10-0 suture can degrade as early as 4 years in children and by 10 years in adults. The 9-0 is much thicker and should have a longer life expectancy. This degradation may not occur with iris fixation. The other tip is to be very careful with the suture placement. With no iris, decentration or tilting of the implant is quite visible. The sutures need to be placed symmetrically, and in some cases they need to be replaced until the lens is centered. A concern in these patients with a 9-mm implant diameter is would the patients be bothered by glare from the peripheral area not covered or blocked by the implant? In my experience with over 100 of these implants, there have been no complaints about this, which initially was a surprise. However, the artificial iris usually reduces visual disturbances so substantially that the recipients are among my happiest patients!

One of the most common problems after iris trauma is rupture of the pupillary sphincter, leaving a pupil diameter of over 9 mm. This can be treated with a purse string suture of 10-0 or 9-0 nylon (Figure 7-2). Use a tapered needle so it does not cut the iris and create more damage. The problem with purse string sutures is that they need many small bites of the iris to look good. They work best through an open sky approach with penetrating keratoplasty. In many of these cases, I implant the Model 311 artificial iris implant, and the cosmetic result is very nice because the color of the patient's iris blends with that of the implant.

In cases of iridodialysis, the dialysis can be repaired with either single- or double-armed 10-0 or 9-0 polypropylene (Figure 7-3). I like to use cutting needles for this because

Figure 7-2. Repair of a ruptured pupillary sphincter with a purse string suture.

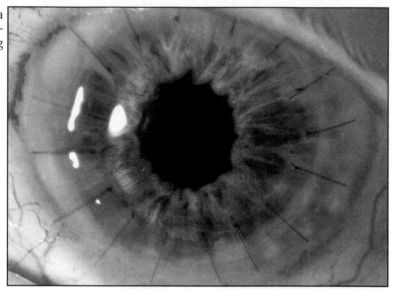

Figure 7-3. Suture repair of iris dialysis following placement of a CTR, phacoemulsification, and IOL implantation in the capsular bag.

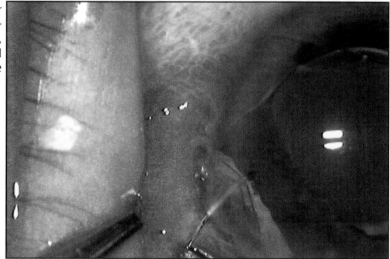

the sutures pass through the sclera. The needle can be placed through the posterior sclera in the area where the attachment should be directed. The needle passes into the eye, catching the peripheral edge of the torn iris with the needle before exiting at the same level of the sclera. An alternative is to make an incision in the peripheral cornea in which one arm of the double-armed suture can be passed into the anterior chamber to grasp the iris and exit out through the appropriate area of the sclera. The second arm does the same maneuver a short distance down the edge of the iris. This provides a mattress suture with better attachment to the iris. With either a single- or double-armed suture, the knot can be rotated into the sclera. When repairing iridodialysis defects like these, assume that the pupil will still be distorted and pulled toward the direction of the repair. This is because the suture bites have to include iris tissue that is normally more centrally located. This causes some shortening of the available iris in that meridian.

PAS and PS should be treated as necessary. Cutting these attachments, especially in cases in which the iris is adherent to the midperipheral or paracentral cornea from a laceration, could produce a larger defect that might require use of an iris implant.

References

1. Price FW, Wellemeyer ML. Transscleral fixation of posterior chamber implants. *J Cataract Refract Surg.* 1995;20:567-573.
2. Price MO, Price FW, Chang DF, Kelley KA, Olson MD, Miller KM. OPHTEC iris reconstruction lens U.S. clinical trial phase I. *Ophthalmology.* 2004;111:1847-1852.
3. Price MO, Price FW, Werner L, Berlie C, Mamalis N. Late dislocation of scleral-sutured posterior chamber intraocular lenses. *J Cataract Refract Surg.* 2005;31:1321-1326.

How Important Is It to Reduce or Eliminate Spherical Aberration and Is There an Advantage to Having Some Present?

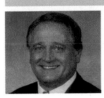

Jack T. Holladay, MD, MSEE, FACS

Spherical aberration is the property of a single spherical surface to refract rays more strongly as one moves from the central optical axis to the periphery (Figure 8-1). The image formed when spherical aberration is present causes a halo (or blur) around the paraxial image (Figure 8-2). The terminology is the same in an optical system with multiple surfaces such as the human eye, which has 4 refracting surfaces (the anterior/posterior cornea and the anterior/posterior crystalline lens). If the system has more optical power laterally from the optical axis toward the periphery, there is positive spherical aberration. If the opposite is true, then it is negative. Spherical aberration is by definition radially symmetric.

Studies measuring ocular spherical aberration of the eye agree on 2 findings. First, there is a great deal of variation in ocular spherical aberration at any age. Second, the average ocular spherical aberration is nearer to zero when people are around 15 to 20 years of age than when they are older. The ocular spherical aberration is the sum of the spherical aberration from the 4 refracting surfaces of the eye.

Studies have demonstrated that the cornea has a stable shape throughout life in the absence of anterior corneal disease such as dry eye or anterior membrane dystrophy.[1] The average spherical aberration of the anterior cornea is +0.270 μm over a 6-mm zone. Glasser and Campbell have shown in vitro that the spherical aberration of the crystalline lens increases (from negative to positive) as a function of age.[2] Two more recent in vivo

Figure 8-1. This diagram of positive spherical aberration illustrates longitudinal and lateral spherical aberration.

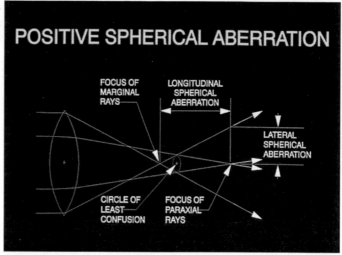

Figure 8-2. Spherical aberration is perceived as halos around lights that cause the symptoms of glare. Increasing amounts of spherical aberration create larger halos.

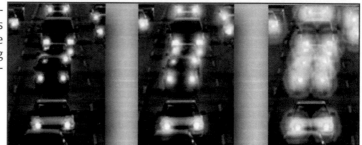

studies[3,4] have shown that the ocular spherical aberration is lowest in people aged 15 to 20. Figure 8-3 is a ray-traced diagram showing that the ocular spherical aberration (entire eye) is nearly zero at around 19 years of age. At this age, the negative spherical aberration of the crystalline lens is almost equal and opposite to the positive spherical aberration of the cornea. Figure 8-4 depicts the spherical aberration in the aging human eye in which the cornea and crystalline lens both have positive spherical aberration.

Is zero the ideal value for spherical aberration? By definition, an aberration reduces the quality of the ocular image. It is true that some aberrations are worse than others. For example, Huber[5] demonstrated better distance vision with similar amounts of with-the-rule versus against-the-rule astigmatism, and Guyton[6] demonstrated that against-the-rule astigmatism was better for near vision. These observations relate to the Arabic alphabet, which has more vertical than horizontal strokes. The common result is that when astigmatism leaves the vertical line of the conoid of Sturm on the retina, the vertical strokes of Arabic letters appear clearest and explain the paradoxical results from Huber and Guyton. Other researchers have demonstrated with image simulation how, together, certain higher-order aberrations can provide clearer images than lower amounts of other aberrations.[7-11] These observations underscore the complex interplay of parameters in the eye that result in our excellent vision.

Spherical aberration does not increase depth of focus. Figure 8-5 depicts the pencil (fan) of rays passing through a 6-mm aperture, coming into focus, and then passing out of focus. Of note, the aspheric intraocular lens (IOL) (no spherical aberration in the system)

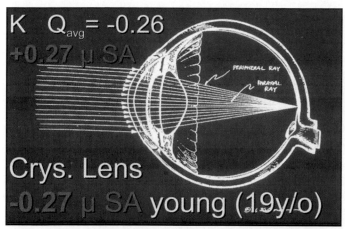

Figure 8-3. The ocular spherical aberration (entire eye) is nearly zero young in life (approximately 19 years of age) because the negative spherical aberration of the crystalline lens is almost equal and opposite to the positive spherical aberration of the cornea.

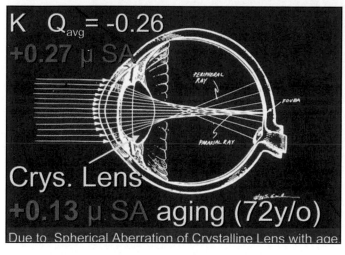

Figure 8-4. The human cornea and crystalline lens both have positive spherical aberration later in life due to the progressive increase in spherical aberration of the crystalline lens with age.

brings rays into a single point of focus, whereas the spherical IOL with spherical aberration does not (forms a blurred circle of least confusion). The only difference between these 2 lenses is at the best focus, where the aspheric surface comes to a single point and the spherical lens does not. At ±0.50 D and beyond, the pencil of light is the same diameter in both the spherical and aspheric IOLs with corresponding, equally blurred circles. There is no difference in the depth of focus, only the clarity of best focus.

The best possible image comes with no spherical aberration because plus or minus spherical aberration yields a blurred halo around the image. However, in presbyopia or pseudophakia with an aspheric monofocal IOL, it may actually be desirable to have a small amount of negative spherical aberration. When negative ocular spherical aberration is present, the power of the eye will effectively increase with pupil constriction, making the near image clearer. Negative spherical aberration still creates a halo, but the near vision with presbyopia is better due to the greater central power. With positive spherical aberration, when the pupil constricts, the power centrally is weaker and actually reduces the quality of the image at near.

Excimer laser surgery has also confirmed these findings. Standard hyperopic treatments induce negative spherical aberration versus positive spherical aberration with

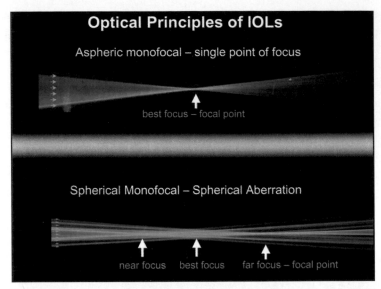

Figure 8-5. The light's path through different IOLs is visualized by projecting a monofocal, green (550-nm) light bundle through a lens positioned in water. The pencil (fan) of rays pass through a 6-mm aperture, come into focus, and then pass out of focus. Of note, the aspheric IOL (no spherical aberration in the system) brings rays into a single point of focus, whereas the spherical IOL with spherical aberration does not (forms a blurred circle of least confusion). The only difference between these 2 lenses is at the best focus, where the aspheric surface comes to a single point and the spherical lens does not. At ±0.50 D and beyond, the pencil of light is the same diameter in both the spherical and aspheric IOLs with corresponding, equally blurred circles. There is no difference in the depth of focus, only the clarity of best focus.

myopic treatments. If patients are emmetropic with presbyopia, the hyperopes with negative spherical aberration will have better near vision than their myopic counterparts with positive spherical aberration. The negative value is also the basis of presbyopic LASIK and Near Vision CK (Refractec, Inc, Irvine, Calif), which produces an exaggeratedly prolate cornea with negative spherical aberration.

What is the optimal ocular spherical aberration target with aspheric IOLs and corneal ablation? From the material already presented, I hope that it is clear that we should target zero spherical aberration in the young individuals with no presbyopia who are scheduled for LASIK or PRK. Because they can accommodate, they will derive no benefit from the introduction of negative spherical aberration. In the presbyope or pseudophake with little or no accommodation, negative spherical aberration may be beneficial if he or she wants to depend less on glasses. If using reading glasses does not bother the patient, then zero spherical aberration is still the best target.

Several clinical studies have demonstrated improved quality with reduced ocular spherical aberration for aspheric IOLs after cataract surgery.[12-15] They have determined the improvement in contrast sensitivity to be approximately 0.3 log units (3 dB) or 40% to 50% improved retinal image contrast. These results are predictable because modern small-incision cataract surgery introduces minimal new corneal aberrations and the optical qualities of IOLs' surfaces far surpass that of the cornea. Measuring the corneal spherical aberration over a 6-mm zone and matching this value with the aspheric IOL with the closest negative spherical aberration is the correct approach. If the surgeon cannot make an exact match, leaving the patient slightly negative is the best choice.

Another consideration that we cannot ignore, when looking at outcome measures such as visual acuity and contrast sensitivity function, is that our visual system includes an optical, sensory, and computer processor. The last of these compares the retinal image to stored images and also enhances the quality of the image. This neural adaptation has both a rapid and a long-term phase that can take up to 1 year. A example is the use of multifocal IOLs, which reduce the contrast of the image by 30% and are associated with halos; however, fewer than 1% of patients notice or are bothered by these effects by 1 year postoperatively. The same is true when the optical system is improved. In the original studies of the TECNIS aspheric IOL, Mester and others showed that the contrast sensitivity function continued to improve from 3 months to 1 year as the brain adjusted to the improved image.[16]

Conclusion

Our refractive surgical goal should be to eliminate or at least reduce all of the optical aberrations of the eye, including spherical aberration. We should remember, however, that it may take 6 months to 12 months of neural adaptation for the patient to fully appreciate and manifest improvement in subjective measures such as visual acuity and contrast sensitivity function. Older presbyopic patients may benefit from a small amount of residual negative spherical aberration in order to achieve better unaided near vision and depend less on glasses. Finally, there is no benefit to leaving any positive spherical aberration in the optical system because it degrades the image and reduces patients' near vision as their pupils constrict.

References

1. Guirao A, Gonzales C, Redondo M, et al. Average performance of the human eye as a function of age in the normal population. *Invest Ophthalmol Vis Science.* 1999;40:203-213.
2. Glasser A, Campbell MCW. Presbyopia and the optical changes in the human crystalline lens with age. *Vision Res.* 1998;38:209-229.
3. Wang L, Santaella RM, Booth M, Koch DD. Higher-order aberrations from the internal optics of the eye. *J Cataract Refract Surg.* 2005;31:1512-1519.
4. Holzer MP, Goebels S, Aufarth GU. Total, corneal and internal aberrations of the human eye. Presented at: Proceedings of the DOC; May 27, 2006; Nuremburg, Germany.
5. Huber C. Planned myopic astigmatism as a substitute for accommodation in pseudophakia. *J Am Intraocul Implant Soc.* 1981;7:244-249.
6. Sawusch MR, Guyton DL. Optimal astigmatism to enhance depth of focus after cataract surgery. *Ophthalmology.* 1991;98:1025-1029.
7. Charman WN. The Charles F. Prentice Award Lecture 2005: optics of the human eye: progress and problems. *Optom Vis Sci.* 2006;83:335-345.
8. Chen L, Singer B, Guirao A, et al. Image metrics for predicting subjective image quality. *Optom Vis Sci.* 2005;82:358-369.

9. Marsack JD, Thibos LN, Applegate RA. Metrics of optical quality derived from wave aberrations predict visual performance. *J Vis.* 2004;4:322-328.
10. Cheng X, Bradley A, Thibos LN. Predicting subjective judgment of best focus with objective image quality metrics. *J Vis.* 2004;4:310-321.
11. Cheng X, Thibos LN, Bradley A. Estimating visual quality from wavefront aberration measurements. *J Refract Surg.* 2003;19:S579-S584.
12. Bellucci R, Scialdone A, Buratto L, et al. Visual acuity and contrast sensitivity comparison between TECNIS and AcrySof SA60AT intraocular lenses: a multicenter study. *J Cataract Refract Surg.* 2005;31:712-717.
13. Kershner RM. Retinal image contrast and functional visual performance with aspheric, silicone, and acrylic intraocular lenses. Prospective evaluation. *J Cataract Refract Surg.* 2003;29:1684-1694.
14. Packer M, Fine IH, Hoffman RS, Piers PA. Prospective randomized trial of an anterior surface modified prolate intraocular lens. *J Refract Surg.* 2002;18:692-696.
15. Packer M, Fine IH, Hoffman RS, Piers PA. Improved functional vision with a modified prolate intraocular lens. *J Cataract Refract Surg.* 2004;30:986-992.
16. Artal P, Chen L, Fernandez EJ, et al. Neural compensation for the eye's optical aberrations. *J Vis.* 2004;4:281-287.

WHAT INTRAOCULAR LENS SHOULD I USE IN THE POSTKERATOREFRACTIVE PATIENT?

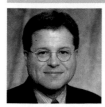

Warren E. Hill, MD, FACS

Since the introduction of radial keratotomy in the United States in 1978, several additional forms of keratorefractive surgery have become popular. David Harmon of *Market Scope* estimates that approximately 1.3 million LASIK procedures will be performed in North America this year. A predictable consequence of such a wide acceptance of keratorefractive surgery over the last 2 decades is that these patients are now coming to cataract surgery in ever increasing numbers.

In the beginning, no one anticipated that unwanted side effects of keratorefractive surgery would include an inability to measure the central corneal power with standard equipment, across the board formula inaccuracies, and the generation of higher-order aberrations (Figure 9-1).

In general, the postkeratorefractive eye can be divided into 3 categories: radial keratotomy, hyperopic laser in situ keratomileusis (LASIK)/photorefractive keratotomy (PRK), and myopic LASIK/PRK. Selecting the correct IOL has three basic components that are carried out differently than would be for a regular IOL power calculation: an estimation of central corneal power, a formula-corrected calculation of IOL power, and selecting the most appropriate IOL type. Combinations of incisional and ablative forms of keratorefractive surgery are beyond the scope of this paper.

Figure 9-1. Zeiss Humphrey ATLAS topographer axial map of an eye with prior radial keratotomy. These eyes are often multifocal and frequently show a dramatic increase in higher-order aberrations, such as positive spherical aberration, Z(4,0).

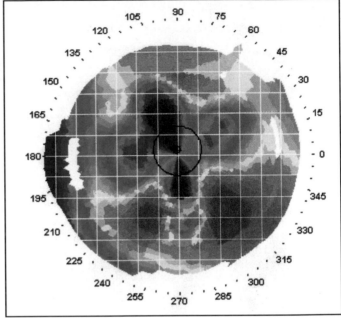

Radial Keratotomy

Radial keratotomy can be approached in a straightforward manner. Because incisional refractive surgery typically exerts an influence on both the anterior and posterior central corneal radii, this allows for a specific form of direct measurement. The 2 methods that we have found to work best are the average of the 1 mm, 2 mm, and 3 mm power values from the Numerical View of the Zeiss Humphrey ATLAS topographer (Carl Zeiss Meditec, Jena, Germany) (Figure 9-2) and the adjusted effective refractive power (EffRPadj) from the Holladay Diagnostic Summary of the EyeSys Corneal Analysis System.[1]

When using a 2-variable, third-generation theoretic formula (Holladay I, SRK/T, or Hoffer Q), the mathematical artifact produced by a very flat central cornea must be removed. Two-variable formulas use only the central corneal power and axial length to estimate the postoperative position of the intraocular lens (IOL). Without some form of special correction, a very low corneal power will often result in the formula assuming that the IOL will be in a more anterior position and call for less IOL power. This effective lens position error will result in unanticipated hyperopia. This effective lens position correction is typically carried out by applying an Aramberri double K method correction or by using the Holladay II formula, which is contained within the Holladay IOL Consultant (Jack T. Holladay, Houston, Tex).[1,2]

Eyes with prior radial keratotomy typically will also have increased higher-order aberrations. While it is not currently possible to correct all of these with an IOL alone, it is possible to offset an elevation in the anterior corneal spherical aberration, Z(4,0). For this, the TECNIS IOL (Advanced Medical Optics, Santa Ana, Calif) with −0.275 µm of negative spherical aberration or the Alcon SN60WF (Fort Worth, Tex) with −0.200 µm of negative spherical aberration can be useful choices. If possible, the surgeon should measure the anterior corneal spherical aberration prior to selecting the most appropriate IOL.

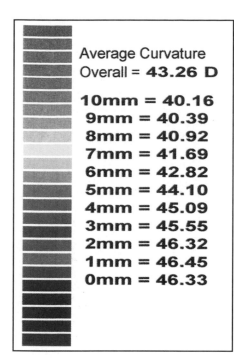

Average Curvature
Overall = **43.26 D**

10mm = 40.16
9mm = 40.39
8mm = 40.92
7mm = 41.69
6mm = 42.82
5mm = 44.10
4mm = 45.09
3mm = 45.55
2mm = 46.32
1mm = 46.45
0mm = 46.33

Figure 9-2. Zeiss Humphrey ATLAS Numerical View power values from an eye with prior hyperopic LASIK. The average of the 1 mm, 2 mm, 3 mm, and 4 mm powers are used in place of keratometry for IOL power calculations.

Hyperopic Laser In Situ Keratomileusis

Eyes that have undergone prior hyperopic LASIK can be treated in much the same way as those with prior radial keratotomy. This is because the ablation pattern is outside the central cornea and typically influences both the anterior and posterior central radii. If the amount of hyperopic LASIK is less than +4.00 D, the average of the 1 mm, 2 mm, and 3 mm power values from the Numerical View of the Zeiss Humphrey ATLAS topographer or the EffRPadj from the Holladay Diagnostic Summary of the EyeSys Corneal Analysis System can be used. For higher powers, Wang, Jackson, and Koch have shown that a small additional correction may be needed.[3]

Again, if using a 2-variable, third-generation formula, an Aramberri double K method correction should be carried out or the Holladay II formula should be used so that the IOL power calculation formula does not miscalculate the effective lens position.

Eyes with prior hyperopic LASIK typically do not show increased spherical aberration because the central cornea has been steepened. If possible, a Z(4,0) value for the anterior cornea should be obtained prior to deciding on which IOL to use. If the Z(4,0) value is low, then a conventional spherical IOL or an aspheric IOL without negative spherical aberration correction, such as the Bausch & Lomb LI61AO (Rochester, NY), would be a reasonable choice. If the measured anterior corneal spherical aberration is close to a median value for the normal population (+0.275 µm) then an IOL such as the Alcon SN60WF would be a good choice. In the rare instance that the anterior cornea spherical aberration Z(4,0) value is markedly elevated, then the AMO TECNIS lens would be appropriate.

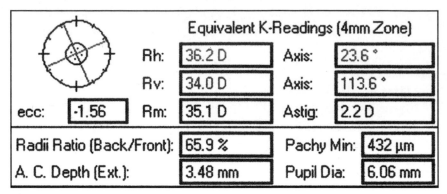

Figure 9-3. Holladay Equivalent K feature of the Oculus Pentacam from an eye with prior myopic LASIK. This method uses data points from both the anterior and posterior corneal radii within a 4-mm zone to calculate a net central corneal power and then converts this information into keratometric diopters.

Myopic Laser In Situ Keratomileusis

Selecting the correct IOL for eyes that have undergone prior myopic LASIK is the most difficult of the 3 common forms of keratorefractive surgery. This is because the anterior radius of the cornea is primarily changed and, at present, there is no consistently reliable methodology available to directly measure the central corneal power.

For estimating the central corneal power, there have been a number of methods proposed, all of which have a limited accuracy. Some are purely historical (Holladay's historical method), some are a combination of historical and objective methods (Masket, Feiz and Mannis, corneal bypass, central corneal power adjustment), while others are purely objective (modified Maloney, Pentacam HEK).[4-7]

What we have found is that the IOL power for the myopic LASIK patient is best determined if calculated by several different techniques, looking for a correlation between historical, historical-objective, and objective methodologies. A summary of the most popular techniques can be found on the Internet at http://www.doctor-hill.com/iol-main/keratorefractive.htm.

The 2 methods that we have found to be the most reliable are Holladay's historical method (provided that the pre-LASIK data is accurate and the post-LASIK refractive information is obtained 4 months to 6 months afterwards) and the Holladay Equivalent K feature of the Oculus Pentacam (Lynwood, Wash) (Figure 9-3).

Again, if using a 2-variable, third-generation formula, an Aramberri double K method correction should be carried out or the Holladay II formula should be used to preclude an unanticipated hyperopic result.

Eyes with prior myopic LASIK will often show an increase in spherical aberration because the central cornea has been flattened. If possible, a $Z(4,0)$ value for the anterior cornea should be obtained prior to deciding which IOL to use. If the $Z(4,0)$ value is close to a median value for the normal population then the Alcon SN60WF would be a good choice. If the anterior corneal $Z(4,0)$ value is elevated, then the AMO TECNIS lens would be more appropriate.

Patients undergoing phacoemulsification with IOL implantation following all forms of keratorefractive surgery will continue to be a challenge until a reliable methodology has been firmly established.

References

1. Aramberri J. Intraocular lens power calculation after corneal refractive surgery: double K method. *J Cataract Refract Surg.* 2003;29(11):2063-2068.
2. Koch D, Wang L. Calculating IOL power in eyes that have had refractive surgery. *J Cataract Refract Surg.* 2003;29(11):2039-2042.
3. Wang L, Jackson DW, Koch, DD. Methods of estimating corneal refractive power after hyperopic laser in situ keratomileusis. *J Cataract Refract Surg.* 2002;28:954-961.
4. Masket S, Masket SE. Simple regression formula for intraocular lens power adjustment in eyes requiring cataract surgery after excimer laser photoablation. *J Cataract Refract Surg.* 2006;32(3):430-434.
5. Wang L, Booth MA, Koch DD. Comparison of intraocular lens power calculations methods in eyes that have undergone LASIK. *Ophthalmology.* 2004;111(10):1825-1831.
6. Holladay JT. Consultations in refractive surgery. *Refract Corneal Surg.* 1989;5:203.
7. Walter KA, Gagnon MR, Hoopes PC, Dickenson PJ. Accurate intraocular lens power calculation after myopic laser in situ keratomileusis bypassing corneal power. *J Cataract Refract Surg.* 2006;32(3):425-429.

How Do I Perform Cataract Surgery in Eyes With a Phakic Intraocular Lens?

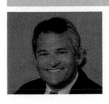

Paul Koch, MD

The best thing about removing a phakic intraocular lens (IOL) in anticipation of cataract surgery is that, unlike inserting one, you do not have to worry about causing a cataract. The strategy is fairly straightforward: remove the phakic lens and then perform the cataract operation.

Having said that, I have removed phakic implants of all 3 types (ie, angle fixated, iris fixated, and sulcus fixated). Each one has its unique features, none of which should be daunting to an experienced cataract surgeon.

There is no angle-fixated phakic lens implant approved for use in the United States, but there are several in use internationally. Most have a polymethylmethacrylate (PMMA) optic between 5 mm and 6 mm, so you will need an incision of at least that width for removal.

The hard part is that the difference between an angle-fixated phakic IOL and an angle-fixated pseudophakic lens is that the former has a convex iris alongside the haptic. I have examined several patients with this type of lens and almost every one had at least a little synechia in the angle. This means that the first step is to analyze the angle to determine whether the IOL will come out easily or whether synechiolysis is needed first (Figures 10-1 to 10-3).

If there are no synechiae, all you have to do is make a 6-mm incision, remove the phakic IOL, suture the incision to 3 mm or so, and then perform your regular phacoemulsification and lens implant procedure.

If there are synechiae, you have to assess whether you think you can break them simply by gently rotating the IOL or by pulling gently on it. If that is not going to happen

Figure 10-1. An angle-fixated phakic IOL that is well centered with a round pupil. There is no sign that there is anything wrong in the angle.

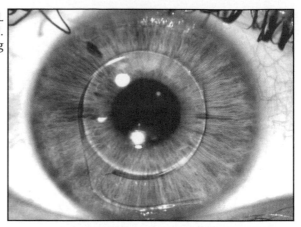

Figure 10-2. This is a goniophotograph of a different eye with an angle-fixated phakic IOL. Early damage can be seen, with depigmentation to the left of center and also on the right, where the iris has chafed against the haptic.

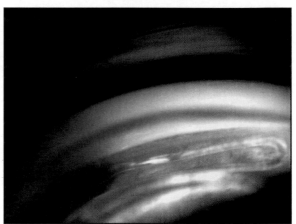

Figure 10-3. Once again, an angle-fixated phakic IOL, but here a cocoon has formed around the haptic. This lens could not be removed easily unless the cocoon was severed under endoscopy.

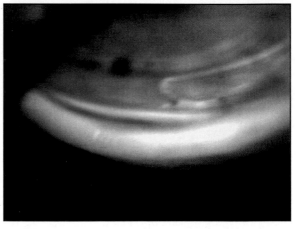

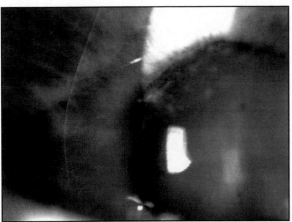

Figure 10-4. This is an iris-fixated phakic IOL in a patient who is very hyperopic. Posterior synechiae have formed and early lens changes are present.

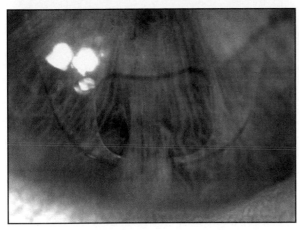

Figure 10-5. An iris-fixated phakic lens can be released easily. While holding onto the lens, gently press a bent needle, a lens hook, or a similar instrument against the peripheral haptic and push the iris out of its grasp.

easily, I suggest using an ophthalmic endoscope to visualize the synechiae and to sever them using a straight 25-gauge needle or a sharp cystotome under direct visualization.

The endoscope will need an incision of about 2.5 mm. The needle will not need its own separate incision; it can be pushed directly into the eye. Using the tip of the needle as a microknife, you can pick, saw, or sever the synechiae in order to free up the haptic. Once it is free, I routinely use a lens hook to rotate the lens a few degrees to be sure there are no remaining adhesions before making my larger incision for removal.

The iris-fixated phakic IOL comes in 2 sizes. All are 8.5 mm in length, but the hyperopic implants and the myopic implants greater than 15 D are 5.0 mm in width. Myopic implants less than 15 D are 6.0 mm in width (Figures 10-4 and 10-5).

I begin these cases by making 2 paracenteses directed toward the enclavation sites and a 3.0-mm phaco incision. Using lens forceps through the phaco incision, I grasp the lens optic while disenclaving the iris from each claw using an enclavation needle or, if you do not have one, a bent 25-gauge needle. If you do not routinely implant these lenses, you will be pleasantly surprised at how easily this is accomplished.

Once the IOL is freed, I enlarge my incision to just slightly larger than the IOL width and remove the lens. I then suture the incision partially closed, leaving a 3.0 mm opening through which I perform my phacoemulsification and foldable lens implant procedure as usual.

Figure 10-6. Sulcus-fixated phakic IOLs sometimes develop anterior lens changes. In this case, the anterior cortical cataract does not involve the optical pathway.

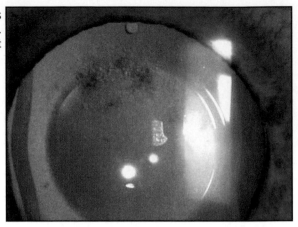

If the lens is sulcus fixated, no special incisions are needed. The standard paracentesis and phaco incisions are made. I use the paracentesis to inject a little viscoelastic under the lens and use a lens hook to pull it into the anterior chamber. These lenses can be removed through a standard phaco incision, after which the cataract operation is performed as usual (Figure 10-6).[1]

You may ask how do you determine the power of the pseudophakic lens that is inserted after removal of the cataract? Can a lens power be determined when a phakic IOL is present during measurements?[2] Usually a pre-phakic IOL biometry exists somewhere. One of the preoperative measurements is the anterior chamber depth, so it is likely that an axial length measurement was done at the same time. If you do not have access to an old axial length, the IOLMaster (Carl Zeiss Meditec, Jena, Germany) is pretty accurate even with a phakic lens in place if you take the measurement with the machine in "phakic" mode. The error in axial length measurement is only about 0.03 mm so you can use that value without modification.[3] There are also theoretical modifications to the axial length reading that might be useful when measuring through thicker, hyperopic lens implants.[4]

References

1. Wiechens B, Winter M, Haigis W, Happe W, Behrendt S, Rochels R. Bilateral cataract after phakic posterior chamber top hat-style silicone intraocular lens. *J Refract Surg.* 1997;13(4):392-397.
2. Pitault G, Leboeuf C, Leroux Les Jardins S, Auclin F, Chong-Sit D, Baudouin C. Optical biometry of eyes corrected by phakic intraocular lenses. *J Fr Ophthalmol.* 2005;28(10):1052-1057.
3. Salz JJ, Neuhann T, Trindade F, et al. Consultation section: cataract surgical problem. *J Cataract Refract Surg.* 2003;29:1058-1063.
4. Hoffer KJ. Ultrasound axial length measurement in biphakic eyes. *J Cataract Refract Surg.* 2003;29(5):961-965.

WHEN SHOULD I USE A TORIC INTRAOCULAR LENS VERSUS ASTIGMATIC KERATOTOMY VERSUS LASER BIOPTICS?

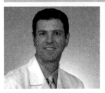

Kerry D. Solomon, MD

Astigmatism treatment has been brought to the forefront of refractive cataract surgery. Surgeons today have numerous options available for the treatment of astigmatism in conjunction with cataract surgery. These options include limbal relaxing incisions (LRIs), toric intraocular lenses (IOLs), and laser vision correction. With the advent of presbyopic IOLs, it is imperative that astigmatism be treated in these patients in order to maximize the patient's visual recovery and minimize dependence on glasses for distance, intermediate, and/or near tasks. In fact, the old adage that less than 1.0 D of astigmatism was clinically acceptable has really been updated. Currently, the majority of refractive cataract surgeons are now aiming to reduce the amount of astigmatism to less than 0.5 D whenever possible.

The treatment of astigmatism as an adjunct to lens-based surgery is based on measured keratometric astigmatism. It is vital that patients be tested with corneal topography to rule out any irregular, asymmetric astigmatism prior to contemplating the use of a presbyopic lens or the management of corneal astigmatism (Figure 11-1). Regular symmetric corneal astigmatism is ideally suited for performing surgical correction. Surgeons should stay away from eyes with irregular, nonorthogonal corneal astigmatism because surgical results are less predictable and underlying forme fruste keratoconus may be present. If a patient has more astigmatism in his or her refraction than that which is measured in his or her cornea, the assumption is that the extra astigmatism is present in the lens, which will be removed. It is, therefore, essential that surgeons focus on assessing the corneal astigmatism as well as the regularity and symmetry of that corneal astigmatism. If patients are not candidates for corneal refractive surgery (LRIs, photorefractive

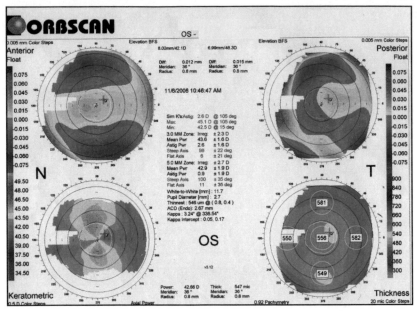

Figure 11-1. Topography of a patient interested in a premium IOL desiring best distance uncorrected vision. This Orbscan topography shows 2.6 D of mostly regular, symmetric corneal astigmatism (anterior curvature, lower left map), relatively centered corneal apex (anterior elevation, upper left map). This is more astigmatism than can be correctable precisely with LRIs. A toric lens (see Figure 11-3) would be the best option for this patient.

keratectomy [PRK], or laser assisted in situ keratomileusis [LASIK]) due to irregular astigmatism, they are not good candidates for presbyopic lenses or refractive cataract surgery, which includes the management of astigmatism. The use of corneal topography has been incredibly helpful in the management and assessment of astigmatism. My preference is one of the newer corneal topographers such as the Pentacam (Oculus, Inc, Lynwood, Wash) or Orbscan (Bausch & Lomb, Rochester, NY), which not only provide curvature data but also elevation data of both anterior and posterior curvatures of the cornea.

Management of Astigmatism in Patients Receiving Presbyopic Intraocular Lenses

For patients receiving presbyopic IOLs, refractive cataract surgeons have 2 options—LRIs or laser bioptics—for treating corneal astigmatism. I use LRIs when the amount of astigmatism is 1.25 D or less. I utilize the Nichamin nomogram as well as the Nichamin blade (Mastel Precision, Rapid City, SD), which is preset at 600 µm. In my experience, LRIs are predictable and relatively easy to perform for 1.25 D or less of corneal astigmatism. These are performed at the same time as the lens surgery (cataract or refractive lens exchange [RLE]). My preference with presbyopic lens implantation is to perform the LRIs at the beginning of the lens extraction surgery.

The technique of LRIs is really quite basic. The axis of the steep meridian is marked in accordance with the Nichamin nomogram. The diamond knife, which is preset at 600 µm, is placed vertical to the corneal curve (tangential) and allowed to sit in place for 1 second to 2 seconds. The LRI is then created by pushing the blade away from the surgeon while the blade is gently rotated in the fingers, similar to rotating a pencil, to remain circumferential with the limbus. As has been described by Dr. Nichamin, the LRI should be located just inside of the corneal vasculature. For LRIs I prefer the use of the fixation ring, which provides excellent control of the eye as well as a nice "guard" to help create a consistent, curvilinear LRI. Any additional "touch-ups" or enhancements after surgery are performed with laser vision correction.

For presbyopic IOL patients with more than 1.25 D of corneal astigmatism, I do not attempt to treat these with LRIs. Instead, patients are notified in advance that their astigmatism will be treated with laser vision correction (PRK or LASIK) following their presbyopic IOL implant. My rationale for performing laser vision correction for astigmatism greater than 1.25 D is quite simple. In my hands, the reliability and accuracy of the treatment is greater with laser vision correction than it is with LRIs. Even though Dr. Nichamin has used LRIs to treat 2.0 D or more of astigmatism, and this is certainly an option if you choose to do so, I still prefer laser vision correction.

LASIK and PRK are both viable options for the treatment of astigmatism[1]; I prefer LASIK. First, I create the corneal flaps using the femtosecond laser (IntraLase [IntraLase Corp, Irvine, Calif]) or the mechanical microkeratome (Amadeus [Advanced Medical Optics Inc, Irvine, Calif]) approximately 1 week to 2 weeks before the cataract or lens exchange surgery. Biometry measurements are obtained prior to the creation of the LASIK flaps and corneal topography is obtained before and after creation of the flap in order to determine that the cornea is stable and ready to undergo cataract surgery. My preference is with the use of the IntraLase because of its reproducibility in creating thin flaps, as well as of the very low incidences of epithelial abrasions.

Once the refraction is stable following the cataract surgery or RLE, the patient is brought to the laser suite. The previously created LASIK flaps are lifted, and the LASIK procedure is performed to treat any residual spherical refractive error (myopia or hyperopia), as well as the pre-existing astigmatism. There are 2 advantages to creating the flaps preoperatively. First, there is a higher level of comfort in knowing that the flap has been created and suction has been placed on the eye before the creation of a clear corneal incision. Second, rather than waiting 3 months to 4 months for the clear corneal incision to be stable enough to perform keratorefractive surgery, previously created flaps can readily be lifted 2 weeks to 4 weeks after lens-related surgery once the refraction is felt to be stable.[2]

As an alternative to LASIK, patients with residual astigmatism can be treated with PRK postoperatively. There are various indications for choosing PRK over LASIK, with the most common being thin corneas. Additionally, PRK has been less associated with the induction of dry eye syndrome, to which cataract patients may already be more prone. PRK surgery can be performed weeks to months after surgery once the refraction is considered stable.

One question that has been raised is whether customized laser vision correction (wavefront) surgery should be performed in the setting of presbyopic lenses. Currently, most surgeons are simply performing conventional surgery for the treatment of myopic or hyperopic astigmatism following presbyopic surgery. Whereas some international and US refractive cataract surgeons have reported good results using wavefront techniques, excellent outcomes have also been reported with conventional techniques. I prefer conventional techniques at this time.

Management of Astigmatism in Patients Receiving Monofocal Intraocular Lenses

The treatment of astigmatism in patients who are not receiving presbyopic IOLs is somewhat different. Toric IOLs are another modality that can be used to treat regular, symmetric astigmatism. Currently, 2 toric IOLs are available for commercial use. The STAAR Toric IOL (STAAR Surgical Company, Monrovia, Calif) with cylindrical powers of 2.0 D and 3.5 D can correct 1.4 D and 2.3 D of astigmatism at the corneal plane, respectively. The AcrySof Toric IOL (Alcon Laboratories, Inc, Fort Worth, Tex) with cylindrical powers of 1.5 D, 2.25 D, and 3.0 D can correct 1.03 D, 1.55 D, and 2.06 D of astigmatism at the corneal plane, respectively (Figures 11-2 and 11-3). These toric lenses do provide very reliable and predictable treatment of pre-existing astigmatism. Because of the possibility of cyclotorsional rotation, it is important to place reference marks on the eye prior to reclining the patient in the surgical suite. I prefer to mark the eye at the 12:00 position, as well as the 3:00 and 9:00 positions. I then use a degree gauge to mark the steep (+) axis of astigmatism. At the completion of the case, the toric IOL is then rotated into the position such that its astigmatic axis is aligned with the steep axis or meridian of the cornea. The STARR Toric IOL rotates quite readily within the capsular bag. My preference is to have the patient lie flat for 30 minutes at the completion of the case and remain relatively inactive for the first 24 hours after surgery to minimize any immediate rotation of the STARR Toric IOL in the capsular bag. My experience has been that the likelihood of this lens rotating is much less after the first 24 hours to 48 hours.

In my experience, the AcrySof Toric IOL has excellent rotational stability almost immediately from the time of implantation. My preference is to initially orient the lens to within 20 degrees of the steep axis (20 degrees counterclockwise to where the lens will finally rest). This is easily done with a second instrument prior to the unfolding of the haptics once the optic is placed into the capsular bag. With viscoelastic removal, the lens tends to rotate 10 degrees to 20 degrees in the clockwise direction, and any final adjustments can be made with a second instrument to align the lens along the steep axis of the cornea. Once the AcrySof Toric IOL is properly aligned, the lens position is stable long term. I do not require that patients lie flat nor do I restrict their activities when I use the AcrySof Toric IOL.

LRIs or laser vision correction can be combined with a toric IOL for those patients with very large amounts of astigmatism. The advantage of using toric IOLs in these eyes is the excellent clarity and quality of vision that they provide.

IOL surgeons have a variety of options and modalities available to them for the management of pre-existing corneal astigmatism. Now that so many patients are expecting spectacle independence after cataract surgery, LRIs, toric IOLs, and/or laser vision correction are essential tools for maximizing patient satisfaction and achieving success.

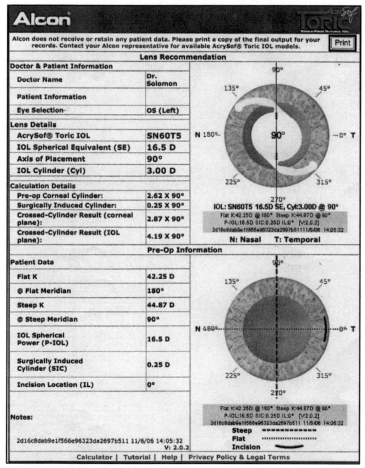

Figure 11-2. The Toric Calculator by Alcon. This calculated 16.5-D AcrySof Toric lens (SNT5) oriented at 90 degrees would be appropriate to reduce the 2.6 D of pre-existing corneal astigmatism as well as the 0.25 D of surgically induced astigmatism from the clear corneal wound.

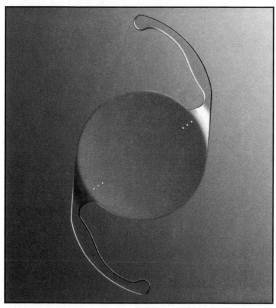

Figure 11-3. Shows the single piece AcrySof toric IOL with the natural chromophore. Note the dotted hash marks near the optic-haptic junction outlining the axis of astigmatism. (Photo provided by Alcon Laboratories, Inc.)

Acknowledgment

I would like to acknowledge the help of Luis E. Fernandez de Castro, MD in writing this chapter.

Supported in part by NIH/NEI grant EY-014793 (vision core) and an unrestricted grant to MUSC-SEI from Research to Prevent Blindness, New York, NY.

References

1. Zaldivar R, Davidorf JM, Oscherow S, et al. Combined posterior chamber phakic intraocular lens and laser in situ keratomileusis: bioptics for extreme myopia. *J Refract Surg.* 1999;15:299-308.
2. Güell JL, Gris O, Muller A, Corcostegui B. LASIK for the correction of residual refractive errors from previous surgical procedures. *Ophthalmic Surg Lasers.* 1999;30:341-449.

MY ASTIGMATIC KERATOTOMY RESULTS ARE UNPREDICTABLE. HOW CAN I IMPROVE THEM?

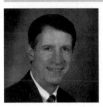

R. Bruce Wallace III, MD, FACS

Limbal relaxing incisions (LRIs) are probably the friendliest and most cost-effective refractive procedures we can offer our patients. There is no expensive laser involved, no central cornea or intraocular trauma, and perforations are rare in healthy corneas. So why is it that many cataract surgeons are not yet using LRIs? Some of us are not convinced that they are reliable, especially if, after purchasing the special instruments, the initial results were disappointing. For many, just the awkwardness of incisional corneal surgery along with an uncomfortable change in routine for surgeon and staff has placed LRIs in a negative light. Yet, judging by the swell in attendance at teaching events like Skip Nichamin's LRI wet labs at the last few American Academy of Ophthalmology and American Society of Cataract and Refractive Surgeons meetings, LRIs are growing rapidly in popularity.

We owe a great deal of thanks to early pioneers who promoted the benefits of combining astigmatic keratotomy with cataract surgery many years ago. A partial list would include Drs. Gills, Hollis, Osher, Maloney, Shepherd, Koch, Thornton, Gayton, Davison, and Lindstrom. Dr. Robert Osher has advocated peripheral relaxing keratotomy at the time of cataract surgery since 1983, learning the principles of the technique from Dr. George Tate.[1]

I have had the pleasure of teaching LRI techniques with Drs. Nichamin, Maloney, Dillman, and many others for over 10 years. During these training sessions, I have learned the steps necessary to convince cataract surgeons that LRIs can be an important part of refractive cataract surgery. Before a cataract surgeon transitions to the routine use of LRIs, he or she must:

* Understand the benefits
* Be confident in the "system" of treatment
* Be confident with his or her technique

Treatment Systems

A systematic approach to LRI use improves results. Gills, Lindstrom, Nichamin, and myself have developed a number of LRI nomograms. I first used Dr. Nichamin's excellent nomogram and then modified it to slant more toward one incision for lower levels of cylinder (Tables 12-1 and 12-2). Since we make our incisions so far in the corneal periphery, paired incisions were not found to be as important for postoperative corneal regularity as traditional astigmatic keratotomy made at the 7-mm optical zone (OZ). An advantage of Nichamin nomograms and their modification is that treatment is planned in degrees of arc rather than cord length. Degree measurements are universally more accurate due to the fact that corneal diameters vary and the fact that we make arcs and not straight line incisions.

For lower levels of astigmatism (less than 2.0 D), selecting the axis of cylinder can be challenging.[2] I look at all axis measurements but usually select ones from computerized corneal topography. Sometimes, especially with smaller cylinder corrections, there is poor correlation of the axis as determined by refraction, K readings, and topography. Many times when I encounter this situation with first eyes for cataract surgery, I will postpone the LRI and measure the cylinder postoperatively. If there is visually disturbing postoperative astigmatism, I will perform LRIs centered on the axis of the postoperative refraction the same day the patient returns for cataract surgery in the fellow eye. Residual astigmatism in the first eye also alerts me to consider an LRI in the second eye.

Questions arise concerning intraocular lens (IOL) power modifications with LRIs. With low to moderate levels of cylinder (0.50 to 2.75), corneal "coupling" equalizes the central cornea power so there is less chance the IOL power selection will be inaccurate. Longer LRI incisions for higher cylinder (>3.0 D) may create a radial keratotomy (RK)-like flattening effect and produce unwanted postoperative hyperopia. Increasing the IOL power by 0.5 D to 1.0 D may be necessary in these cases.

Instrumentation

Simplification of instruments and techniques improves efficiency and comfort with the procedure. There are many excellent LRI instrument sets available from Mastel, Rhein, Katena, ASICO, and others. I designed the "Wallace LRI Kit" with Duckworth & Kent (Hertfordshire, England). This kit includes:
* Pre-set single foot plate trifacet diamond knife (600 µm)
* Mendez axis marker
* 0.12-caliber forceps

The trifacet diamond is less likely to chip. The Mendez marker has actual numbers on the dial to help guide the surgeon to the proper axis mark. (This orientation guide is

<u>Table 12-1</u>

The "NAPA" Nomogram: Nichamin Age and Pachymetry-Adjusted Intralimbal Arcuate Astigmatic Nomogram

With-the-Rule (Steep Axis 45 degrees to 145 degrees)				
Preoperative Cylinder (Diopters)	Paired Incisions in Degrees of Arc			
	20 to 30 years old	31 to 40 years old	41 to 50 years old	51 to 60 years old
0.75	40	35	35	30
1.00	45	40	40	35
1.25	55	50	45	40
1.50	60	55	50	45
1.75	65	60	55	50
2.00	70	65	60	55
2.25	75	70	65	60
2.50	80	75	70	65
2.75	85	80	75	70
3.00	90	90	85	80
Against-the-Rule (Steep Axis 0 degrees to 40 degrees/140 degrees to 180 degrees)				
Preoperative Cylinder (Diopters)	Paired Incisions in Degrees of Arc			
	20 to 30 years old	31 to 40 years old	41 to 50 years old	51 to 60 years old
0.75	45	40	40	35
1.00	50	45	45	40
1.25	55	55	50	45
1.50	60	60	55	50
1.75	65	65	60	55
2.00	70	70	65	60
2.25	75	75	70	65
2.50	80	80	75	70
2.75	85	85	80	75
3.00	90	90	85	80

When placing intralimbal relaxing incisions following or concomitant with radial relaxing incisions, total arc length is decreased by 50%.

Created by and used with permission of Louis D. "Skip" Nichamin, MD of Laurel Eye Clinic, Brookville, Pa.

Table 12-2

Limbal Relaxing Incisions

Instruments

- Diamond knife: Trifacet 600 µm preset depth, single foot plate
- Marker: Mendez axis ring
- Forceps: 0.12 caliber

Procedure

- Place axis ring around limbus.
- Mark axis with forceps.
- Mark limits of intended incision(s) with forceps.
- Remove axis ring.
- Dry marks with cellulose sponge.
- Fixate globe with forceps.
- Perform incision(s), direct toward fixation.

Nomogram

Assuming all cataract incisions are performed temporally and are relatively astigmatically neutral:

For With-the-Rule and Oblique Astigmatism

Astigmatism (in diopters)	40 to 50 years old	50 to 60 years old	60 to 70 years old	70 to 80 years old	80+ years old
1.00 to 1.50	60 degrees[1]	50 degrees[1]	50 degrees[1]	40 degrees[1]	30 degrees[1]
1.50 to 2.00	70 degrees[1]	70 degrees[1]	70 degrees[1]	60 degrees[1]	60 degrees[1]
2.00 to 2.50	60 degrees[2]	60 degrees[2]	60 degrees[2]	70 degrees[1]	70 degrees[1]
2.50 to 3.00	70 degrees[2]	70 degrees[2]	70 degrees[2]	60 degrees[2]	60 degrees[2]
3.00 to 4.00	80 degrees[2]	80 degrees[2]	80 degrees[2]	70 degrees[2]	70 degrees[2]

For Against-the-Rule Astigmatism

Astigmatism (in diopters)	40 to 50 years old	50 to 60 years old	60 to 70 years old	70 to 80 years old	80+ years old
1.00 to 1.50	60 degrees[1]	50 degrees[1]	40 degrees[1]	40 degrees[1]	30 degrees[1]
1.50 to 2.00	70 degrees[1]	60 degrees[1]	60 degrees[1]	60 degrees[1]	40 degrees[1]
2.00 to 2.50	60 degrees[2]	80 degrees[1]	80 degrees[1]	70 degrees[1]	60 degrees[1]
2.50 to 3.00	70 degrees[2]	70 degrees[2]	70 degrees[2]	60 degrees[2]	60 degrees[2]
3.00 to 4.00	80 degrees[2]	80 degrees[2]	80 degrees[2]	70 degrees[2]	70 degrees[2]

[1] denotes 1 incision
[2] denotes 2 incisions

When using nomogram, if age/astigmatism at dividing point:
- Choose the shortest incision length
- Choose 1 incision over 2 incisions

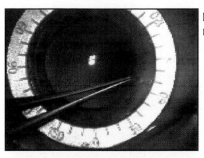

Figure 12-1. Marking the astigmatic axis with a Mendez ring.

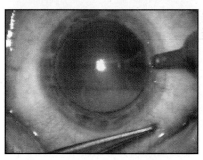

Figure 12-2. LRI placed 1.0 mm to 1.5 mm from the surgical limbus.

valuable because the biggest fear—besides a perforation—is placing the incision in the wrong axis.) All of these instruments are made of titanium to increase longevity.

Patient Counseling

Similar to preoperative discussion of the new refractive IOLs, informing patients about the option of surgical treatment for astigmatism has become commonplace in many cataract practices. We start by describing the optical disadvantages of astigmatism and the relative effectiveness and low risk surrounding LRIs. In the United States, when charging Medicare patients for an additional out-of-pocket fee for LRIs, an advanced beneficiary notice (ABN) should be filed.

Technique

A surgeon's LRI technique will vary depending on the instruments used for the procedure. The routine I use with the Duckworth & Kent instruments is as follows:

* Make the LRIs before making the phaco incision, but after wetting the cornea.

* Mark the axis (Mendez ring and 0.12 forceps).

* Mark the incision borders (Mendez ring and 0.12 forceps).

* Fixate the globe (0.12 forceps).

* Advance the knife toward fixation (usually toward the surgeon).

Try to insert the knife into the peripheral corneal dome (approximately 1.5 mm from the actual limbus) as perpendicular as possible (Figures 12-1 and 12-2). Maintain this blade orientation and with moderate pressure complete the LRI by "connecting the dots" on the cornea and twirling the knife handle to make an arcuate incision using the limbus as a template.

Postoperative Care

For many years, we added a nonsteroidal anti-inflammatory drug (NSAID) (Acular, Allergan, Inc, Irvine, Calif) to our postoperative cataract surgery regimen to offer corneal analgesia. We now use an NSAID (Acular LS, Allergan, Inc) routinely for all cataract surgery patients, preoperatively and postoperatively, mainly to help reduce inflammation and the incidence of cystoid macular edema. A topical fourth-generation fluoroquinolone (Zymar, Allergan, Inc) and steroid (PredForte, Allergan, Inc) are also part of my medication routine for cataract surgery. We do not patch the eye after LRIs but do apply povidone-iodine 5% on the cornea preoperatively and immediately postoperatively.

Measuring Results

A number of methods are available to measure our results with LRIs. Newer computer software includes postoperative astigmatic analysis. Surgically induced refractive change and vector analysis are often used to demonstrate astigmatic change. A simpler way to follow results is just to measure the amount of postoperative cylinder at any axis. If a patient has <0.75 D of postoperative astigmatism, he or she is likely to be happy with his or her results.

The Future of Limbal Relaxing Incisions

Like phacoemulsification, LRI instruments and techniques will continue to evolve. As we follow LRI results with imaging such as sophisticated corneal topography and wavefront aberrometry, modifications such as adjustments in blade depth and optic zone diameter will help us improve. Competition with toric IOLs and combinations of bioptics with corneal laser and light adjustable IOLs may reduce LRI popularity. Regardless, any improvement in methods to reduce unwanted astigmatism will continue to be an important part of successful refractive cataract surgery.

References

1. Osher RH. Consultations in refractive surgery. *J Refract Surg.* 1987;3(6):240.
2. Wallace RB. On-axis cataract incisions: where is the axis? *1995 ASCRS Symposium of Cataract, IOL and Refractive Surgery Best Papers of Sessions.* 1995;67-72.

FOR HOW LONG SHOULD TOPICAL ANTIBIOTICS AND NONSTEROIDAL ANTI-INFLAMMATORY DRUGS BE USED BEFORE AND AFTER CATARACT SURGERY?

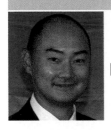

Francis S. Mah, MD

First and foremost, when discussing antibiotic prophylaxis for cataract surgery, it must be stressed that the use of the antiseptic povidone-iodine 5% solution in the conjunctival cul-de-sac prior to surgery is the cornerstone of endophthalmitis prophylaxis.[1]

There is no consensus on which antibiotic to use or the method of application surrounding cataract surgery; however, there is general agreement that perioperative antibiotics are the standard of care.[2-6] Since there are no prospective, randomized clinical trials regarding when to start antibiotic prophylaxis, we will defer to the plethora of studies done by our general surgery colleagues.[7-10] The studies in general surgery have shown that the most efficacious time to use antibiotics is no more than 1 hour prior to surgery; 30 minutes prior to starting the incision is the optimal time to begin intravenous antibiotic prophylaxis.[10] Many ophthalmic surgeons point to studies done by Frank Bucci[11] and Christopher Ta,[12] which show a decrease in periocular bacterial flora as the rationale for using preoperative topical antibiotics 1 day to 7 days prior to cataract surgery. Although this is surrogate evidence that there may be prophylactic efficacy to this strategy, other reasons may make this strategy useful (eg, teaching patients to use medications from a reusable dropperette). Since there is no extra cost to the health care system, one bottle will typically last long enough for effective cataract surgery prophylaxis, and since there most likely is no harm being done, as long as the patient is using the medication in the manner accepted by the Food and Drug Administration (FDA), the strategy of using preoperative

Figure 13-1. Recommended topical antibiotics.

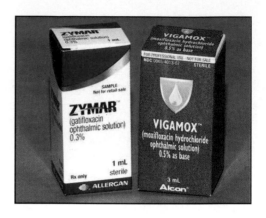

antibiotics day(s) prior to cataract surgery can be an acceptable means for prophylaxis, if not yet proven. The reason I do not use antibiotics day(s) prior to surgery stems from my fear that the patient may not follow instructions that he or she is typically given week(s) before surgery. Were patients to use the antibiotic for weeks prior to surgery or use varying doses, resistant bacteria may be selected prior to surgery. Furthermore, a patient may lose the bottle or use the entire bottle, adding to the cost of surgery.[13]

Again, since the ophthalmic peer-reviewed literature is of no help in terms of the optimal time to end postoperative use of antibiotics for the purpose of prophylaxis, we will turn to the general surgery literature, which shows that the benefits of postoperative intravenous antibiotics last for the first 12 hours, 24 hours maximum.[7-10] The general indication in ophthalmic surgery is to use topical antibiotics until the epithelium is healed, roughly 3 days to 10 days.[2,4] Due to the use of topical steroids following cataract surgery, which are not typically used following general surgery procedures, I think it is prudent to use topical antibiotics until the epithelium is intact following cataract surgery. Although it is typical to taper steroids and other anti-inflammatory medications, it is important not to taper antibiotics due to the real risk of developing and selecting for bacteria that are resistant.[14] Therefore, the recommendation is to start using topical antibiotics at least 30 minutes to 1 hour prior to surgery and continue the medication at full FDA dosage until the epithelium is healed, roughly 3 days to 10 days, without tapering the antibiotic.

Which antibiotic to use is even less clear. Several caveats to use while deciding which antibiotic include peak concentrations (Cmax) in the ocular tissues and the minimum inhibitory concentration (MIC) of the key bacteria that cause endophthalmitis. Other characteristics may be considered such as spectrum of coverage, cidal versus static mechanism, biocompatibility, cost, etc, but the main characteristics that define antibiotic efficacy are Cmax and MIC.[15] Today in ophthalmic surgery, fluoroquinolones generally have the desirable combination of the lowest MICs and the highest concentrations in ocular tissues when used topically.[15] Currently, among the fluoroquinolone class, gatifloxacin and moxifloxacin are the most potent (lowest MICs) and reach the highest concentrations in the cornea and the anterior chamber (highest Cmax).[15] It is my opinion that cataract surgeons should be utilizing 1 of these 2 agents for perioperative cataract surgery prophylaxis (Figure 13-1).

Recently, a large European collaboration has created earnest discussion among cataract surgeons regarding the future of prophylaxis.[2] The study found a significant reduction in the rates of endophthalmitis when using intracameral cefuroxime at the conclusion of

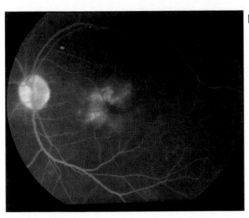

Figure 13-2. CME.

surgery. As of this moment, the final manuscript has not been published, but ongoing critiques of the study include the use of levofloxacin as the topical antibiotic, cefuroxime as the intracameral agent, the relatively high rate of endophthalmitis seen in this study, and the potential long-term and short-term adverse events, including toxic anterior segment syndrome from administering intracameral antibiotics that are not commercially prepared.[2] Intracameral antibiotics may be the future of cataract surgery endophthalmitis prophylaxis, but important questions must be addressed before they become the standard of care.

Unlike the use of topical antibiotics, the perioperative use of topical nonsteroidal anti-inflammatory drugs (NSAIDs) surrounding cataract surgery has been studied in prospective trials. Regarding miosis prevention, management of postoperative pain, and control of postoperative inflammation, the peer-reviewed literature is unanimous in showing that topical NSAID used 3 days prior to surgery is superior to 1 day, which is superior to the day of surgery.[16-18]

Postoperative length of therapy for an NSAID is less elucidated in the literature. The general opinion is that topical NSAIDs should be used for 3 weeks to 4 weeks following cataract surgery, but this is not based on efficacy studies.[16-18] If we look at the fact that cystoid macular edema (CME) (Figure 13-2) has a peak incidence of 4 weeks to 6 weeks following routine uncomplicated surgery, then it makes sense that the NSAID should be used at least 6 weeks to 8 weeks to cover the high-risk period. In those patients at higher risk such as diabetics, uveitics, vasculopaths, and complicated surgery patients, to name a few, the use of prophylactic NSAIDs should be used for at least 8 weeks to 12 weeks. The dosing should never exceed the FDA recommended frequency, and the eye should be monitored carefully in all patients with extended NSAID use beyond 4 weeks due to the risk of corneal and scleral melts. The risk of these postoperative melts is highest in neurotrophic keratopathy patients, severe dry eye patients, and other patients with moderate to severe ocular surface disease such as blepharitis and meibomitis.[16-18]

Regarding the NSAID of choice, as of this writing, there are many head-to-head studies trying to determine if there are any significant differences between commercial products. The peer-reviewed literature shows the efficacy of diclofenac, ketorolac 0.5%, bromfenac 0.09%, and nepafenac 0.1% in the management of postcataract surgery inflammation and pain.[16-18] Diclofenac and ketorolac have been shown to be efficacious in the management of CME in the literature. The newest NSAIDs, bromfenac and nepafenac, are reportedly more potent and are reportedly more bioavailable after topical dosing. Nepafenac is the only pro-drug.[16-18] Until there is prospective data showing differences between the available NSAIDs, it makes sense that the pain management, CME prevention, and anti-inflammatory efficacy are class effects. Several key differences are the dosing (twice a day to four times a day), the formulations (solution versus suspension), and the rate of burning and stinging in the FDA trials (0% to 40%).

The recommendation for topical NSAID use for all patients undergoing cataract surgery (except those mentioned at high risk for sclero-corneal melts) is 3 days before surgery optimally, day of surgery minimally, and at the FDA-approved dose extended to 6 weeks to 8 weeks following surgery. For those at high risk for CME following cataract surgery, the use of NSAIDs should start at least 3 days prior to surgery and be continued for at least 8 weeks to 12 weeks.

References

1. Speaker MG, Menikoff JA. Prophylaxis of endophthalmitis with topical povidone-iodine. *Ophthalmology.* 1991;98:1769-1775.
2. Barry P, Seal DV, Gettinby, G, et al. ESCRS study of prophylaxis of postoperative endophthalmitis after cataract surgery. *J Cataract Refract Surg.* 2006;32(3):407-410.
3. Jensen MK, Fiscella RG. Comparison of endophthalmitis rates over four years associated with topical ofloxacin vs ciprofloxacin. (Poster) Association for Research in Vision and Ophthalmology, May 2002, Ft. Lauderdale, Fla.
4. Masket S. Preventing, diagnosing, and treating endophthalmitis. *J Cataract Refract Surg.* 1998;24:725-726.
5. Fisch A, Salvanet A, Prazuck T and The French Collaborative Study Group on Endophthalmitis. Epidemiology of infective endophthalmitis in France. *Lancet.* 1991;338:1373-1376.
6. Montan PG, Wejde G, Setterquist H, Rylander M, Zetterstrom C. Prophylactic intracameral cefuroxime: evaluation of safety and kinetics in cataract surgery. *J Cataract Refract Surg.* 2002;28:982-987.
7. Bratzler DW, Hunt DR. The surgical infection prevention and surgical care improvement projects: national initiatives to improve outcomes for patients having surgery. *Clin Infect Dis.* 2006;43:322.
8. Zanetti G, Platt R. Antibiotic prophylaxis for cardiac surgery: does the past predict the future? *Clin Infect Dis.* 2004;38:1364.
9. Finkelstein R, Rabino G, Mashiah T, et al. Vancomycin versus cefazolin prophylaxis for cardiac surgery in the setting of a high prevalence of methicillin-resistant staphylococcal infections. *J Thorac Cardiovasc Surg.* 2002;123:326.
10. Bratzler DW, Houck PM, et al. Antimicrobial prophylaxis for surgery: an advisory statement from the national surgical infection prevention project. *Clin Infect Dis.* 2004;38:1706.
11. Bucci FA Jr. An in vivo study comparing the ocular absorption of levofloxacin and ciprofloxacin prior to phacoemulsification. *Am J Ophthalmol.* 2004;137(2):308-312.
12. Ou JA, Ta CN. Endophthalmitis prophylaxis. *Ophthalmol Clin North America.* 2006;19(4):449.
13. Ta CN, He L, Nguyen E, De Kaspar HM. Prospective randomized study determining whether a 3-day application of ofloxacin results in the selection of fluoroquinolone-resistant coagulase-negative Staphylococcus. *Eur J Ophthalmol.* 2006;16(3):359-364.
14. Mah FS. Fourth-generation fluoroquinolones: new topical agents in the war on ocular bacterial infections. *Curr Opin Ophthalmol.* 2004;15(4):316-320.
15. Mah FS. New ocular antibiotics. *Ophthalmol Clin N Am.* 2003;16(1):11-27.
16. O'Brien TP. Emerging guidelines for use of NSAID therapy to optimized cataract surgery patient care. *Curr Med Res Opin.* 2005;21(7):1131-1137.
17. Lindstrom R, Kim T. Nepafenac: ocular permeation and inhibition of retinal inflammation: an examination of data and opinion of clinical utility. *Curr Med Res Opin.* 2006;22(2):397-404.
18. McColgin AZ, Heier JS. Control of intraocular inflammation associated with cataract surgery. *Curr Opin Ophthalmol.* 2000;11(1):3-6.

SECTION II

INTRAOPERATIVE QUESTIONS

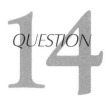

UNDER TOPICAL ANESTHESIA, THE PATIENT IS UNCOOPERATIVE AND COMPLAINING OF PAIN. WHAT SHOULD I DO?

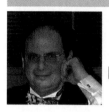

Kenneth J. Rosenthal, MD, FACS

Topical anesthesia can be successfully used in a majority of routine cataract surgical cases. In fact, almost any patient who can have surgery under block anesthesia (peri- or retro-bulbar anesthesia) may also be a suitable candidate for topical anesthesia.[1] When carefully balanced with intravenous (IV) sedation, it can be helpful in maintaining a comfortable surgical encounter. The goal of the topical anesthetic is to ablate pain, while the goal of the IV sedation is to garner the cooperation of the patient. IV sedation should be administered in a titrated dosage so as to relieve anxiety and allow the patient to remain stationary, calm, comfortable, and cooperative without creating obtundation.[2]

The distinction between anesthesia and sedation is important to understand. While some surgeons feel that the complete lack of sensation provided by a regional block may improve patient cooperation, they may sometimes find that the lack of cooperation is behavioral (such as an anxious or controlling personality) and not related to the feeling of pain or other discomfort and that the decision to block the patient did not solve the problem. It has been my experience that with proper patient counseling, both topical and injectable anesthesia are of equal effectiveness with the obvious additional advantage that topical is inherently safer as an anesthetic method.

Topical anesthetic may consist of topical eye drops (eg, 1% to 4% lidocaine, 0.5% tetracaine, or 0.5% proparacaine), topical lidocaine jelly (alone or in combination with a cocktail of mydriatics, which is my preference), or Tetravisc (CYNACON/OCuSOFT,

Table 14-1

Dilation Protocol for Topical Anesthesia

Lidocaine Jelly 2% (20 g/mL) 5 cc
Tropicamide 1% 5 drops
Cyclopentolate 2% 5 drops
Phenylephrine 10% 5 drops
Acular (Allergan, Inc, Irvine, Calif) (ketorolac tromethamine 0.5% ophthalmic solution) 5 drops
Zymar (Allergen, Inc, Irvine, Calif) (gatifloxacin 0.3% ophthalmic solution) 5 drops

0.5 cc is dispensed into the inferior fornix using an aseptic technique and is delivered through a 1-cc tuberculin or insulin-type syringe.

Reprinted with permission of Island Eye Surgicenter, Carle Place, NY.

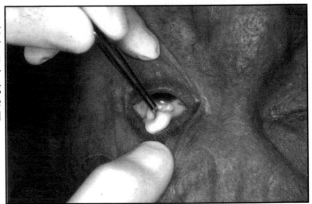

Figure 14-1. Rosenthal deep topical nerve block anesthesia. An anesthetic sponge can be placed in the superior and/or inferior fornices saturated with anesthetic, mydriatics, antibiotics, or nonsteroidal anti-inflammatory drug or combinations thereof to produce a more profound effect than topical application.

Rosenberg, Tex) (0.5% tetracaine gel) (Table 14-1). A pledget or sponge delivery system may be employed when more profound anesthesia is desired.

An example of the use of the sponge as a vehicle to deliver anesthetic to the eye is the Rosenthal deep topical nerve block anesthesia (Figure 14-1),[3,4] which may be delivered by placing a pledget of absorbent surgical sponge soaked with the desired medication in the eyelid fornices. Penetration of the anesthetic may be enhanced by application of pressure to the sponge through the closed lid with a device such as a Honan's balloon. The term *topical anesthesia* is usually understood to encompass the use of intracameral anesthetics (instilled by blunt cannula during surgery) even though it is not applied to the ocular surface, which may be used alone or in combination with topical agents.[5]

The management of a patient who is unstable (ie, "uncooperative and complaining of pain") begins with the preoperative clinical encounter. While the patient's behavior prior to entering the operating room does not always correspond to the surgical encounter itself, the patient's demeanor, level of anxiety, and responses to touching the eyelids during examination may give clues as to how he or she will fare during surgery and may guide the decision as to what depth and type of sedation the patient may require in order to successfully and safely endure the surgical experience.[6,7] The patient should be

counseled to expect to see bright lights, feel pressure in the eye, and be aware of the surgeon touching the eyelids. The patient should be assured that IV sedation will be given
and that he or she will be "relaxed but awake" during the procedure. He or she should
be encouraged to let the surgeon know if he or she feels anxious or restless and should
be assured that the anesthesia care provider will give supplemental sedation to make the
patient comfortable when needed.

Let us consider first the scenario in which the patient confirms that he or she has
bona fide pain. A topical anesthetic can be augmented by adding additional amounts
of the agent used preoperatively or with an intracameral instillation of 1% lidocaine.[5,8]
This technique is used by many surgeons routinely because it provides additional anesthetic effect, has been shown to be nontoxic to the intraocular tissues,[9] and may facilitate
mydriasis. It should be used with caution in patients who have vitreous prolapse or in any
condition in which there is a conduit to the posterior pole because the drug may cause
prolonged (but fully reversible) amaurosis due to absorption by the retina.

If the patient's complaints of "pain" are actually a manifestation of anxiety caused
by feeling an unfamiliar sensation such as pressure, quiet reassurance may be all that is
needed to regain the patient's confidence and cooperation. It is also helpful to keep extra-
neous conversation in the operating room to a minimum, to play music that has a sooth-
ing effect, to occasionally "check in" with the patient to make sure he or she is comfortable, to hold his or her hand (by the circulator or anesthesia care giver, not the surgeon!!),
and to provide the patient with a "progress report" as reassurance that surgery is going
as planned. These techniques may be collectively referred to as "vocal local." In cases
in which these measures do not suffice, carefully titrated additional IV sedation may be
given, keeping in mind that there are wide variations in patients' susceptibility to these
agents and that the elderly are particularly sensitive to small dosage increments.

In cases in which the patient's cooperation cannot be obtained despite having already
administered an optimal dose of sedation, the option to convert to general anesthesia,
when available, should be considered. This extends also to patients who have language
difficulty, are deaf, or who have head or body movement disorders or nystagmus.
Surprisingly, however, many such patients can be successfully managed with a balanced
topical and IV sedation technique, which may ablate the tremor or nystagmus. Language
problems or deafness can often be overcome by appropriate discussion preoperatively.

In cases in which the possibility of requiring general anesthesia is anticipated, I will
make a first attempt by administering topical anesthesia and appropriate sedation. A
general anesthetic is given only if an anxiolytic dosage of sedation is given and the patient
still cannot cooperate.

Even many chronically ill patients can safely undergo a brief general anesthesia but
control of the airway must be maintained. This is safer than resorting to sedating a
patient to the point of obtundation, which may cause acute dementia or agitation. This
often sudden and dreaded event is highly likely to result in a surgical complication.

When general anesthesia is used, it should nonetheless be supplemented with a topical
anesthetic because this will reduce the depth of general anesthetic needed, applying again
the principle that systemic medication is used for behavioral control and the regional
topical anesthetic anesthetizes the eye itself. For brief cases, the safety and postoperative
comfort of general anesthesia can be furthered by the use of laryngeal mask anesthesia
(LMA) (Figure 14-2).[10] Since it is placed in the larynx rather than the trachea, problems

Figure 14-2. The laryngeal mask anesthesia device can be placed in the larynx without a laryngoscope, providing safe, rapid induction of general anesthesia for short cases.

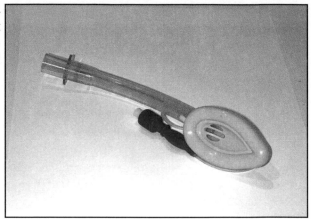

associated with endotracheal intubation (eg, sore throat, potential of bronchial intubation, damage to teeth) can be avoided and it does not require a laryngoscope for placement.

Even complex cases can be managed with a balanced topical anesthetic and IV sedation technique. Topical and intracameral anesthesia are highly effective even when vitrectomy is required, regardless of whether it is performed through the anterior segment or (as is my preference) through the pars plana. The sponge anesthesia method has been shown to be effective for vitrectomy, scleral tunnel, and even extracapsular techniques. In the event that additional local anesthesia is needed, however, conversion to sub-Tenon's anesthesia is easily accomplished and is about as effective as injectable anesthesia with the added benefit that it will ablate any eye movement. There are several variants of this technique: a small conjunctival peritomy is made behind the limbus and a cannula is slipped beneath the conjunctiva, directed posteriorly along the globe, and a bolus of anesthetic is injected. Cannulae designed by Masket, Greenberg, and Fukasaku,[11] to name a few, maximize the delivery of the anesthetic posteriorly, but any blunt-tipped cannula (eg, an olive-tipped cannula) can be used successfully.

Appropriate preoperative evaluation, patient counseling, and a clear understanding of the relationship between anesthesia and systemic sedation will allow a pain-free, comfortable, and anxiety-free experience for most patients. An understanding of the options to supplement or convert anesthetic technique intraoperatively can further enhance the effectiveness of this technique.

References

1. Claoue C. Simplicity and complexity in topical anesthesia for cataract surgery [comment]. *J Cataract Refract Surg.* 1998;24(12):1546-1547.
2. Rosenthal KJ. Complications of topical anesthesia. In: Fishkind W, ed. *Complications in Phacoemulsification.* Stuttgart, NY: Georg Thieme Verlag; 2002.
3. Rosenthal KJ. Deep, topical, nerve-block anesthesia. *J Cataract Refract Surg.* 1995;21(5):499-503.
4. Rosenthal KJ. Deep topical nerve block anesthesia. In: Davis D, ed. *Ophthalmology Clinics of North America.* Philadelphia: WB Saunders; 1996.
5. Crandall AS, Zabriskie NA, Patel BC, et al. A comparison of patient comfort during cataract surgery with topical anesthesia versus topical anesthesia and intracameral lidocaine. *Ophthalmology.* 1999;106(1):60-66.

6. Dinsmore SC. Approaching a 100% success rate using topical anesthesia with mild intravenous sedation in phacoemulsification procedures. *Ophthalmic Surg Lasers.* 1996;27(11):935-938.

7. Dinsmore SC. Drop, then decide approach to topical anesthesia [see comments]. *J Cataract Refract Surg.* 1995;21(6):666-671.

8. Gills JP, Cherchio M, Raanan MG. Unpreserved lidocaine to control discomfort during cataract surgery using topical anesthesia. *J Cataract Refract Surg.* 1997;23(4):545-550.

9. Gills JP. Corneal endothelial toxicity of topical anesthesia [letter; comment]. *Ophthalmology.* 1998;105(7):1126-1127.

10. Poloch A, Romaniuk W, Jalowiecki P, et al. [Evaluation of the usefulness of the laryngeal mask for general anesthesia in eye microsurgery—preliminary results]. *Klin Oczna.* 1996;98(1):45-49.

11. Fukasaku H, Marron JA. Pinpoint anesthesia: a new approach to local ocular anesthesia. *J Cataract Refract Surg.* 1994;20(4):468-471.

How Should I Proceed if I Made a Poor Clear Corneal Incision?

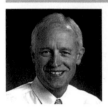

Randall J. Olson, MD

Is it good enough or not? It certainly hydrated just fine; however, there is definitely a tear in the wound edge. What should I do? We have all been there, and yet poorly constructed incisions increase the risk of endophthalmitis. At the Moran Eye Center, University of Utah, we went from an incidence of 1 in 1200 to 1 in 400 with clear corneal surgery.[1] Furthermore, a prospective randomized trial[2] and a study of Medicare data[3] showed clear corneal incisions can be associated with increased endophthalmitis. Because many others have not experienced this same trend, the difference is likely associated with how we handle marginal wounds.

We showed that a leaky clear corneal wound on the first day increases the risk of endophthalmitis 44-fold![1] This is not a situation we ever want to be in and, therefore, we need to recognize and know how to deal with the marginal wound.

I believe that an appropriate clear corneal incision has a length into the eye that is at least two-thirds of its width at all points along the incision. These incisions first close mechanically as the intraocular pressure seals an appropriately constructed internal lip. Corneal endothelial pumping then reinforces this seal and is therefore integral to providing a proper fluid barrier.

To minimize incision complications, such as endophthalmitis, it is important to recognize a marginal wound and to close or reinforce it with a suture. For example, marginal wounds result if the keratome is tilted as it passes through the cornea. If the plane of the blade is not coming in parallel to the corneal plane, then one side will cut out and the other side often will cut back into the conjunctiva. This is especially true when diamond blades are used (Figure 15-1). Therefore, as the keratome is advancing into the cornea,

Figure 15-1. In this incision, the keratome has cut into the cornea on one side and into the conjunctiva on the other side because the blade was slightly tilted as it entered the eye. The side into the cornea is now the most likely place for the wound to leak and conjunctival ballooning is likely from cutting into conjunctiva on the opposite side.

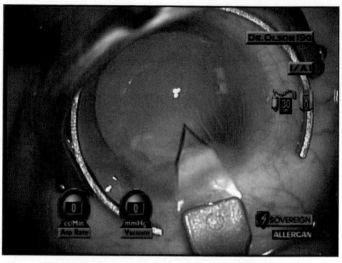

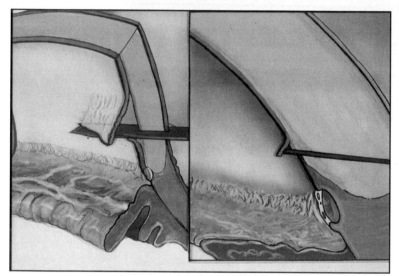

Figure 15-2. Descemet's tear. As a dull blade enters the eye, Descemet's membrane resistance to penetration can result in a small peripheral single tear. Now with the endothelial cells on Descemet's pulled away from the stroma, there is no endothelial pump to help further seal the wound. Any instrumentation can cause this problem as it enters the eye. (From Fishkind WJ, ed. *Complications in Phacoemulsification: Avoidance, Recognition, and Management.* New York, NY: Thieme Medical Publishers; 2002. Reprinted with permission.)

take a moment to monitor how cleanly both sides are advancing and adjust the blade path accordingly. Another cause of a marginal wound is a small Descemet's detachment (Figure 15-2). Extra scrutiny is required to see the telltale sign of a torn Descemet's membrane flapping in the current as you inflate the eye through the side-port incision. If Descemet's membrane is not apposed against the wound, then the endothelial pump is ineffective. Finally, beware of wounds that are so small that they are internally torn by the instruments that are passed through them. When an otherwise well-constructed incision leaks profusely, consider this possibility. Although stromal hydration may close this kind of wound, it only lasts 10 minutes to 15 minutes and leakage is therefore still a concern.

If my incision is marginal or poorly constructed, I place a single 10-0 nylon suture. I want to see a watertight closure without stromal hydration in order to have full confidence in the incision closure. I remove this 10-0 nylon at the 1-week postoperative visit and have never had a problem with continuing leakage at that time. An ounce of prevention is worth a pound of cure and, indeed, we were able to improve our endophthalmitis rate from 1 in 400 to better than 1 in 1200 mainly by suturing marginal wounds.

Other issues to consider in regard to increased risk of endophthalmitis from clear corneal incisions are as follows:

*   Wounds that tend to fish-mouth (keratoconus, previous corneal transplant, or corneal scars). I feel these incisions also deserve a suture.

*   Capsular rupture or zonular breakage (13.7-fold increased risk of endophthalmitis[1]). These eyes are already at increased risk of endophthalmitis, and the incision must be 100% secure.

What about patients with previous radial keratotomy (RK)? If I can work between RK incisions, then a clear corneal wound is not a problem; however, if this is not possible, I do a small peritomy without cautery and start my incision about 1 mm posterior to the conjunctival insertion with a small scleral groove. The entry into the chamber is in the normal fashion; however, I look for an area that is well healed. That small strip of sclera keeps the peripheral edge from separating and as long as I am careful about not having the bottle too high and using moderate flow, I have not seen problems with this.

Another potential problem associated with clear corneal incisions is inadvertently nicking the conjunctival insertion. With infusion, Tenon's acts like a subconjunctival sponge that can potentially create 360 degrees of conjunctival ballooning. Such exasperating ballooning causes irrigation fluid to pool over the cornea, which in turn compromises the intraocular view. In this case, making a conjunctival incision and a small tenonectomy just behind the corneal incision and then "milking" some of the fluid out is very effective. To prevent this from occurring, we must be sure to monitor the posterior edges of our advancing keratome to ensure that one side is not incising the conjunctival insertion.

Conclusion

If you suspect a marginal cataract incision, you should take the time to place a corrective suture because this can reduce the risk of endophthalmitis. Our experience at the Moran Eye Center supports this idea.

Acknowledgment

Supported in part by a grant from Research to Prevent Blindness, Inc, New York, NY, to the Department of Ophthalmology and Visual Sciences, University of Utah.

References

1. Wallin T, Parker J, Jin Y, Kefalopoulos G, Olson RJ. Cohort study of 27 cases of endophthalmitis at a single institution. *J Cataract Refract Surg.* 2005;31:735-741.
2. Nagaki Y, Hayasaka S, Kadoi C, et al. Bacterial endophthalmitis after small incision cataract surgery: effect of incision placement and intraocular lens type. *J Cataract Refract Surg.* 2003;29:20-26.
3. West E, Behrens A, McDonnell P, et al. The incidence of endophthalmitis after cataract surgery among the U.S. medical population increased between 1994 and 2001. *Ophthalmology.* 2005;112:1388-1394.

16

WHAT SHOULD I DO IF THE CHAMBER IS SO SHALLOW THAT IT DOES NOT DEEPEN MUCH WITH VISCOELASTIC?

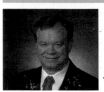

Johnny Gayton, MD

Anatomically, narrow angles are a worldwide problem, but they are especially common in rural Georgia. Many of the eyes with narrow angles are hyperopic. This high incidence of hyperopia led me to develop the piggyback lens technique in an effort to better rehabilitate these eyes following lens surgery.

Patients with narrow angles generally develop increasing narrowing of the angle with age. I explain this to the patient by describing that the lens grows in circumference by adding rings like a tree. In people with narrow angles, this increase in circumference encroaches on the already limited anterior segment space. Many patients with narrow angles will ultimately develop angle closure. Dr. Harry Quigley estimates that angle-closure glaucoma will account for 26% of all glaucoma by the year 2010.[1,2] It accounts for almost half of the blindness caused by glaucoma today.[1,2] After witnessing several cases of blindness, even in patients who had laser iridotomies, I concluded that the best treatment for narrow angles is lens removal.

Lens removal has been my treatment of choice for narrow angles or impending phacomorphic glaucoma for the past 18 years. A recent study reported in the January 2006 issue of the *Journal of Cataract and Refractive Surgery* concluded that lens extraction reduced intraocular pressure in patients with narrow angles regardless of whether they had been treated by laser iridotomy.[3] The patients treated with cataract extraction alone did not need additional medication, whereas those who had been previously treated with laser iridotomy frequently still needed medication. A study performed by Dr. Sturmer showed 108 eyes with relative anterior microphthalmos (ie, a normal axial length with a small anterior segment) that did well with cataract surgery alone.[4]

Figure 16-1. Narrow angle as observed by slit lamp. (Reprinted with permission from Ledford JK, Sanders V. *The Slit Lamp Primer, Second Edition.* Thorofare, NJ: SLACK Incorporated; 2005.)

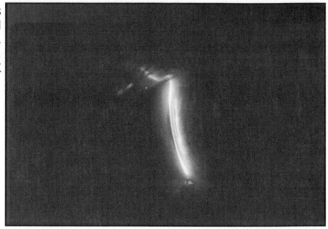

Laser iridotomy does not prevent the increasing lens size from causing encroachment on the anterior chamber angle, and it has its own set of complications, including transient intraocular pressure rise, iridocyclitis, hyphema, cataract formation, endothelial cell loss, and synechia formation. It is much more likely that a patient will need an additional procedure if his or her narrow angle is treated with laser iridotomy rather than lens removal.[5] Lens removal also offers the advantage of improving the patient's uncorrected vision and preventing further maturation of the lens, resulting in the difficult removal of a hard nucleus in a shallow anterior chamber. When we make the diagnosis of a narrow angle by slit-lamp examination (Figure 16-1) or gonioscopy, we advise the patient of his or her options: observation, laser iridotomy, or lens extraction. Patients who choose observation are required to sign a consent that discusses their increased risk of angle closure. We also have a letter that we send to patients with anatomically narrow angles who have refused treatment.

I feel topical anesthesia is usually best in patients with narrow angles since a periocular injection increases orbital pressure, making the surgery more difficult. Prior to making the incision, the intraocular pressure is checked by digital palpation. If the intraocular pressure is elevated, the patient is given IV mannitol. If this does not adequately soften the eye, we perform a vitreous tap by inserting a 27-gauge needle through the pars plana. Enough fluid is aspirated to soften the eye. I do a lot of these cases and rarely do a vitreous tap. It is very important to construct a proper wound in the narrow-angle patient. I attempt to make at least a 2-mm corneal tunnel in order to decrease the likelihood of iris prolapse. Viscoelastic is then used to fill the anterior chamber. The side-port incision is angled so that any instrument inserted through the side port can easily reach the area of the cataract incision, where it can be used to help resolve any potential iris prolapse. If the iris should start knuckling toward the wound, immediately stop irrigation and depress either the cannula or the surgical instrument being used downward, allowing egress of fluid from behind the iris. If this does not take care of the iris prolapse, I insert a cannula through the side-port incision and place a small amount of viscoelastic over the iris in an attempt to tamponade it into position. If iris prolapse continues to be a significant problem, I close the wound with a shoestring 10-0 nylon and move to another location. I feel that an extra corneal wound is less risky than dealing with iris prolapse throughout a case, which will cause iris atrophy and potentially damage the iris sphincter.

A 5-mm capsulorrhexis is carefully performed. If this attempts to run radially, a second instrument is placed through the side-port wound and the nucleus is pushed slightly posterior as the capsulorrhexis is completed. Gentle hydrodissection is performed with 1% unpreserved lidocaine on a Chang cannula (Rumix International, St. Petersburg, Fla). It is important to avoid excessive hydrodissection, which can cause iris prolapse. In some patients, the angle is so narrow that I debulk the lens with the phacoemulsification handpiece prior to performing hydrodissection. Debulking the lens gives more room to work and aspirates some of the viscoelastic, making a corneal burn unlikely. In narrow-angle cases, it is important to use viscoelastic that does not easily leave the anterior chamber and retains space well. I have had excellent results using Viscoat (Alcon, Fort Worth, Tex), DiscoVisc (Alcon, Fort Worth, Tex), and Healon 5 (Advanced Medical Optics, Santa Ana, Calif). Many patients with narrow angles have coexisting corneal guttata or Fuchs' dystrophy; therefore, protection of the corneal endothelium with a highly retentive viscoelastic is imperative. The nucleus is dissembled using a combination of chopping techniques. I have found the Chang chopper (Katena Products Inc, Denville, NJ) to be very helpful during this stage. Its sharp end can be used for a quick chopping technique especially in patients with hard nuclei. The curved end can be used for dividing and chopping and as a manipulator. After removing the nucleus, gentle hydrodissection of the subincisional epinucleus and cortical material is performed using an irrigating J cannula. The epinucleus and cortical material are then removed. Viscoelastic is instilled and the intraocular lens is inserted. If one implant can adequately correct the patient, I prefer a single implant to a piggyback. If the patient needs too much power to be corrected by one implant, my current technique is to insert an acrylic lens into the capsular bag and insert a silicone lens into the ciliary sulcus. I place most of the power in the acrylic lens, so that the silicone lens can be as thin as possible, decreasing the likelihood of pupillary block. Many eyes with narrow angles do not have proportional anatomy. This does influence intraocular lens calculation. The Holladay IOL Consultant (Jack T. Holladay, Houston, Tex) improves accuracy by including anterior chamber depth and corneal diameter in the calculations.

References

1. Lin S. Angle closure: more than meets the eye. *Rev Ophthalmol.* 2006;13(6):82-84.
2. Quigley HA, Broman AT. The number of people with glaucoma worldwide in 2010 and 2020. *Br J Ophthalmol.* 2006;90:253-254.
3. Imaizumi M, Takaki Y, Yamashita H. Phacoemulsification and intraocular lens implantation for acute angle closure not treated or previously treated by laser iridotomy. *J Cataract Refract Surg.* 2006;32:85-90.
4. Sturmer J, Kniestedt C, Meier F. Cataract and combined cataract/glaucoma surgery as intraocular pressure reducing in eyes with relative anterior microphthalmos. *Klin Monatsbl Augenheilkd.* 2005;222(3):206-210.
5. Lim L, Hussain R, Gazzard G, et al. Cataract progression after prophylactic laser peripheral iridotomy: potential implications for the prevention of glaucoma blindness. *Ophthalmology.* 2005;112:1355-1359.

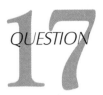

QUESTION

17

MY CAPSULORRHEXIS FLAP TORE RADIALLY. HOW SHOULD I PROCEED?

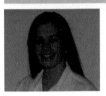

Rosa Braga-Mele, MEd, MD, FRCSC

Continuous curvilinear capsulorrhexis is one of the most important steps in successful phacoemulsification and intraocular lens insertion.[1] It is important to proceed carefully during this step and avoid an errant capsulorrhexis tear.

Avoidance of a radial tear is key. The main cause of an errant capsular tear is a shallowing of the anterior chamber, with a subsequent excursion of the rhexis peripherally along the path of least resistance. Thus, one should ensure that the anterior capsule is flat during the entire capsulorrhexis procedure. The capsule is kept flat by making certain that the anterior chamber is filled with either a dispersive or cohesive viscoelastic. If needed, one should refill the anterior chamber with viscoelastic as necessary. If the chamber is particularly shallow, one may opt for a viscoadaptive viscoelastic such as Healon 5 (Advanced Medical Optics, Santa Ana, Calif) to aid in deepening the chamber. When performing a capsulorrhexis with Healon 5, the rhexis tends to want to turn inward and thus an errant tear is less likely to occur. One must also ensure that the speculum or drape does not cause any unnecessary pressure on the globe, thereby shallowing the chamber. It is important to regrasp the rhexis frequently, at least every 90 degrees, and ensure that one's grasp is close to the edge of the flap. Viscoelastic can also be used to direct the leading capsular flap into an optimal direction and position.

If the lens is hypermature or white, one should use a capsular staining dye to ensure visibility of the anterior capsule during the procedure. There have been many staining techniques described,[2] but my preference is to use trypan blue in a small aliquot "painted" directly onto the anterior capsule underneath some viscoelastic. Also, if there appears to be any positive pressure produced by the contents of a hypermature lens, it is beneficial

Figure 17-1. Errant radial tear occurring.

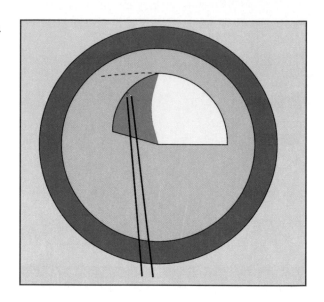

to decompress the lens with a 25-gauge needle inserted into the anterior capsule prior to beginning a capsulorrhexis in order to avoid the "Argentinean flag sign" (capsule tearing centrally end to end).[3] One can also tamponade the capsule with the use of Healon 5 in this case.

If the rhexis should start to run radially (Figure 17-1), then I suggest taking a deep breath and injecting more viscoelastic into the anterior chamber either through the main incision or the side-port incision. While placing the viscoelastic and with other instrument insertions, take extreme care not to shallow the chamber any further by exerting undue pressure on the incisions. If one cannot visualize the edge of the tear, then one can use a light pipe placed at the limbus that is directed across the surface of the capsule to provide enhanced contrast. Alternatively, one can use trypan blue to stain the edge of the capsule[4] at this point in the procedure to aid in visualization.

If you are now able to visualize the leading edge of the rhexis, you can proceed in 1 of 2 ways:

1. If the tear is small and has not gone out too far, then the flap can be grasped in its turned-over position and redirected centrally by turning it acutely 90 degrees from the edge of the flap. This can be a difficult maneuver through a small incision due to restricted movement of the wrist.

2. If the tear is more radial, you can use viscoelastic to reflatten or unfold the flap so that it lies flat on the surface of the lens back over into its original position (Figure 17-2). Then place the capsulorrhexis forceps at the edge of the flap/tear and pull initially circumferentially and then straight toward the center of the lens.[5,6] This will ensure that the edge of the tear will be propagated toward the center and away from the radial direction even for those tears that have almost reached the zonules. Again, it cannot be emphasized enough that it is important to have a flat anterior capsule and lens surface; therefore, viscoelastic reinjection is important. Once the edge of the rhexis is in a safe position, one can proceed with the rhexis in the usual manner.

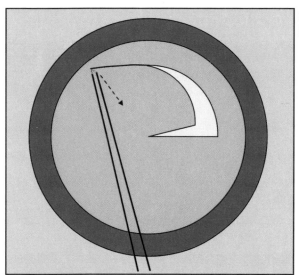

Figure 17-2. Unfold flap to lie flat on the lens and pull centrally.

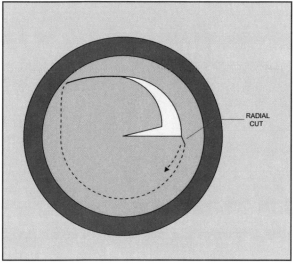

Figure 17-3. Restarting a rhexis with a radial cut.

RADIAL
CUT

If the tear has proceeded radially to the point of no return past the zonules, then one must rethink the procedure. Either restart the rhexis at the original starting point by creating a radial cut at the edge of the rhexis and then proceeding with the rhexis in the opposite direction to meet the errant tear (Figure 17-3) or—at this point—perform a can-opener capsulotomy for the remaining capsule. There has also been some literature that describes suturing an aberrant tear, which can restore the strength and elasticity of the rhexis.[7] At this point, it is probably safest to flip the nucleus into the anterior chamber and proceed with phacoemulsification in the anterior chamber. Alternatively, one could consider converting to a large incision extracapsular procedure if the nucleus is extremely dense.

Acknowledgment

I would to thank Ted Christakis (medical student, University of Toronto) for his help in literature searches and his creation of the figures present in this paper.

References

1. Gimbel HV, Neuhann T. Development, advantages, and methods of the continuous circular capsulorrhexis technique. *J Cataract Refract Surg.* 1990;16:31-37.
2. Dada V, Sharma N, Sudan R, et al. Anterior capsule staining for capsulorrhexis in cases of white cataract: comparative clinical study. *J Cataract Refract Surg.* 2004;30:326-333.
3. Chan D, Ng A, Leung CK, Tse RK. Continuous curvilinear capsulorrhexis in intumescent or hypermature cataract with liquefied cortex. *J Cataract Refract Surg.* 2003;29:431-434.
4. Waard P, Budo C, Melles G. Trypan blue capsular staining to find the leading edge of a lost capsulorrhexis. *Am J Ophthalmol.* 2002;134:271-272.
5. Little B. Tear out retrieval, a mystery unfolds. ASCRS Film Festival. 2006.
6. Little BC, Smith J, Packer M. Little capsulorrhexis tear out rescue. *J Cataract Refract Surg.* 2006;32:1420-1422.
7. Kleinmann G, Chew J, Apple DJ, Assia EL, Mamalis N. Suturing a tear of the anterior capsulorrhexis. *Br J Ophthalmol.* 2006;90:423-426.

DESPITE ATTEMPTING HYDRODISSECTION, I CANNOT ROTATE THE NUCLEUS. HOW SHOULD I PROCEED?

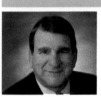

William J. Fishkind, MD, FACS

The hydrosteps consist of hydrodissection and hydrodelineation. To answer this question, I would first like to review how to properly perform cortical cleaving hydrodissection.

Cortical Cleaving Hydrodissection

For cortical cleaving hydrodissection,[1,2] I prefer a standard 27-gauge cannula attached to a 3-cc syringe filled with balanced salt solution (BSS). However, any cannula designed for this function is first placed just superior to the anterior capsular edge and then withdrawn slightly and dropped just beneath the anterior capsule. The tip is then advanced and elevated under the anterior capsule until it is halfway between the anterior capsular rim and the capsular bag equator. This assures a peripheral position between the cortex and anterior capsule. The tip of the cannula is elevated enough to just tent the anterior capsule. A steady, firm stream of BSS is then injected. The stream of BSS passes anteriorly toward the anterior capsule, around the proximate equator, then behind the posterior pole of the cataract, and around to the opposite equator, around the opposite equator, and into the anterior chamber. Slight depression of the shaft of the cannula against the posterior lip of the incision during fluid injection allows excess fluid to pass through the incision, preventing overinflation of the anterior chamber. This is especially important if a dispersive ophthalmic viscosurgical device (OVD) is used. The end point of fluid injection is the visualization of the nucleus floating anteriorly. Gentle posterior pressure on the nucleus

Figure 18-1. Illustration of the nuclear, cortical, capsular bag connections, which must be lysed to allow unrestrained rotation of the cataract. (From Fishkind WJ, ed. *Complications in Phacoemulsification: Avoidance, Recognition, and Management.* New York, NY: Thieme Medical Publishers; 2002. Reprinted with permission.)

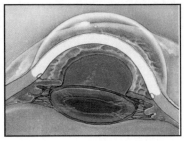

will effectively push fluid sequestered behind it around the equator. The hydrodissection should be performed first on one side and then again in a location 180 degrees opposite. If performed effectively, the cortex is separated or cleaved from the capsule, allowing free rotation of the endonucleus, epinucleus, and cortex as a unit within the capsular bag. This will lyse all nuclear, cortical, capsular bag connections (Figure 18-1).

CONVENTIONAL HYDRODISSECTION

Standard hydrodissection is performed in a similar manner except the cannula is placed within the substance of the cortex. This produces a cleavage plane within the cortex. Consequently, part of the cortex remains adherent to the capsular bag and part is adherent to the endonucleus.

Hydrodelineation

Immediately following hydrodissection, the same cannula is moved to the paracentral zone of the nucleus. It is then embedded within the nuclear substance. The cannula tip is moved to and fro to create a track within the nuclear material. BSS is then injected slowly into the bulk of the nucleus. The BSS will find the surgical plane at the junction of the epinucleus and endonucleus and will separate them. Even after adequate hydrodelineation, the endonucleus will not rotate independently of the adjacent epinucleus and cortex.

Hydrodelineation is necessary to perform those phaco procedures requiring lens disassembly, such as phaco chop.

Why Perform Cortical Cleaving Hydrodissection?

There are several reasons to switch from conventional hydrodissection to cortical cleaving hydrodissection. The latter technique is performed more peripherally in order to cleave cortex from the capsular bag. The surgeon can then separate the endonucleus from the epinucleus and cortex via hydrodelineation. These 2 maneuvers permit phacoemulsification to be performed in 2 stages. The endonucleus is removed first, followed by the epinucleus and adherent cortex. As the cataract becomes more mature, the epinucleus becomes increasingly important as a protective shell during nucleofractis. It will prevent sharp fragments of nucleus from tearing the posterior capsule, especially if postocclusion surge should occur. Once the endonucleus is emulsified, the cataract will lose its rigidity.

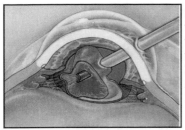

Figure 18-2. The phaco tip has aspirated cortex adherent to the capsular bag. The adherent cortex does not separate from the bag. Pulling on the endonucleus to rotate it or aspirating the endonucleus will result in breaking adjacent zonules. (From Fishkind WJ, ed. *Complications in Phacoemulsification: Avoidance, Recognition, and Management.* New York, NY: Thieme Medical Publishers; 2002. Reprinted with permission.)

It can easily be elevated to the plane of the iris for emulsification using lower power and vacuum settings to minimize surge. Lysing the cortical-capsular bag connections allows more complete cortical removal during phaco. This minimizes irrigation and aspiration (I&A) time and lessens stress to the zonules and ciliary body during I&A.

In the presence of a torn posterior capsule, cortical cleaving hydrodissection facilitates the removal of cortex during I&A without enlarging the tear since the cortex is not adherent to the capsular bag. If the patient's zonules are weak, cortical cleaving hydrodissection makes it easier to remove the epinucleus and cortex and reduces the risk of tearing more zonules and disrupting the capsular bag.

Adherent Epinucleus and Cortex

The above steps should ensure a freely rotating nucleus 95% of the time. If the nucleus does not turn freely, then the hydrodissection was incomplete. The surgeon should repeat the procedure. In fact, hydrodissection can be repeated at any time. For example, if hydrodissection needs to be repeated, phaco can be interrupted after the initial chop in vertical chopping, or after the nucleus is cracked in a stop-and-chop technique. The crack in the nucleus presents an exit path for the BSS injection, which will complete the hydrodissection by flowing under and around the heminucleus. Occasionally, with a small amount of OVD to maintain the anterior chamber, 2 instruments can be introduced to work against the counter pressure of the vitreous to tire iron the nucleus and free it from the capsular bag.[3] If the nucleus does not rotate freely, divide-and-conquer and horizontal chopping techniques are contraindicated. The rotational maneuvers necessary for divide and conquer may result in stressed and torn zonules or a tear in the capsular bag (Figure 18-2). Trying to place the chopper around the equator of the lens when it is still attached to the capsular bag may have a similar result.

If repeated or complete hydrodissection is impossible, the surgeon must exercise greater care during phacoemulsification in order to avoid stressing the zonules. Approaching the equatorial cortical material too closely may result in phacoing through the equatorial bag (Figure 18-3). If complete hydrodissection appears impossible and the nucleus will not freely rotate, then—as previously described—vertical chopping is the technique of choice. Eventually, enough endonucleus will be removed so that the remaining endonucleus and epinucleus will become mobile. Exercise caution in this situation because an immobile nucleus may indicate an occult tear in the capsular bag or weak zonules.

Figure 18-3. With continued aspiration, the equatorial capsular bag will be engaged and torn. (From Fishkind WJ, ed. *Complications in Phacoemulsification: Avoidance, Recognition, and Management.* New York, NY: Thieme Medical Publishers; 2002. Reprinted with permission.)

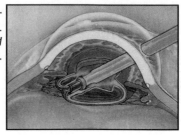

Intentional Incomplete Hydrodissection

Occasionally, the conscious decision not to complete hydrodissection is indicated. A nick in the anterior capsule or a discontinuous capsulorrhexis (eg, one that extended toward the equator and had to be finished from the other side) is a good reason not to complete hydrodissection. Injecting too much fluid might cause a capsular tear that extends to the equator or (worse) into the posterior capsule. Another reason that surgeons might hesitate to complete hydrodissection is poor visualization due to a small pupil. A posterior polar cataract also calls for special hydrodissection maneuvers (see Question 23).

Some might forego complete hydrodissection in cases of pre-existing zonular weakness caused by trauma or pseudoexfoliation. Although it is difficult to hydrodissect and fully rotate the nucleus in these cases, I believe they actually require extra hydrodissection. Mackool capsular bag support hooks, Cionni rings (Morcher GmbH, Stuttgart, Germany), or Ahmed capsular tension segments all enhance successful hydrodissection in these eyes. If the surgeon can carefully employ multiple small hydrodissection injections until the nucleus is completely free, then removing the endonucleus, epinucleus, and cortex will be easier and less traumatic to the zonules.

Conclusion

Cortical cleaving hydrodissection and hydrodelineation are important early steps of cataract surgery. Performed carefully, successful completion leads to an easier surgical procedure. Encountering an adherent nucleus, which will not rotate, is a salvageable problem if recognized. Carefully repeating hydrodissection, or performing a vertical chopping technique, will generally overcome the problem.

References

1. Fishkind WJ, ed. *Complications in Phacoemulsification: Avoidance, Recognition, and Management.* New York, NY: Thieme Medical Publishers; 2002.
2. Fine IH. Cortical cleaving hydrodissection. *J Cataract Refract Surg.* 1992;18:508-512.
3. Chang DF. *Phaco Chop: Mastering Techniques, Optimizing Technology, and Avoiding Complications.* Thorofare, NJ: SLACK Incorporated; 2004.

FOLLOWING HYDRODISSECTION, THE IRIS IS PROLAPSING AND THE GLOBE IS VERY FIRM. HOW SHOULD I PROCEED?

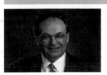

I. Howard Fine, MD

Following hydrodissection, the eye suddenly becomes very firm and the iris prolapses. In this situation, one must highly suspect that it was the hydrodissection itself that caused the problem; however, it is necessary to rule out other sources.

External forces have to be considered and are quickly assessable. If injection anesthesia has been used, there could be an orbital hemorrhage. This can be ruled out easily by gentle displacement of the globe to show that the orbit is indeed not firm. The lock mechanism on the speculum could suddenly have released, resulting in partial closure of the lid with forcing of the speculum blades against the globe, or the patient's lids may be strong enough to overcome the less firm opening of the wire-lid speculums. In addition, anything that can lead to Valsalva's maneuvers must be considered. Pain, extreme anxiety, cough or cough suppression, and a full bladder causing the patient to strain are all possible causes. Each of these Valsalva's maneuvers can lead to impairment in venous drainage from the globe and the orbit. Communicating with the patient immediately by asking what is wrong and recommending normal breathing can quickly alleviate this problem.

Intraocular sources of pressure must be considered. A choroidal effusion or a suprachoroidal hemorrhage will frequently be detected by either a loss of red reflex or by a dark shadow appearing within the red reflex. A fundus contact lens in the operating microscope, or an indirect ophthalmoscope, can be used to immediately assess the posterior segment of the eye and rule in or out this diagnosis. If the eye is extremely firm and the view is poor, one may wish to proceed rapidly with a B-scan. Generally, there is increasing data that a sclerotomy does not alleviate the problem but may exacerbate the problem with excessive bleeding increasing the danger to the eye.

Figure 19-1. The hydrodissection cannula is used through the same paracentesis to sweep posterior to the internal lip of the incision to reposit the iris.

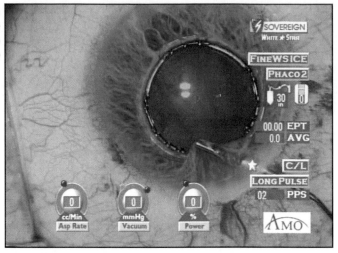

The most likely cause in the present situation, however, is overhydration during the course of hydrodissection. Cortical cleaving hydrodissection is a maneuver that I first described in 1991[1] and involves tenting the anterior capsule with a cannula peripheral to the capsulorrhexis margin and gently injecting fluid into the capsular bag external to the cortex. The fluid goes around the lens and becomes loculated in the capsule behind the lens as the fluid reaches the forniceal capsular-cortical connections, which disallow its emergence from the retrolenticular space. This is observable by a forward movement of the lens, which makes the capsulorrhexis enlarge. The hydrodissection should be stopped at that point and the cannula should depress the lens posteriorly, which would increase intracapsular pressure and force posteriorly loculated fluid to come forward around the equator of the lens, rupturing the capsular-cortical connections and flowing out of the capsulorrhexis. This is observed by an immediate return to the previous, smaller size of the capsulorrhexis, as well as radial striations on the anterior surface of the lens as cortical fibers are washed centrally. In order for the cortical cleaving hydrodissection to work, there has to be an intraoperative capsular block syndrome, which is cured by decompression of the capsule by downward pressure on the lens.

In the instance in which the eye is firm and the iris is prolapsing, the hydrodissection cannula should be used through a paracentesis to decompress the lens, while at the same time exerting pressure on the posterior lip of the paracentesis incision to allow egress of fluid and viscoelastic. Once that is done, the hydrodissection cannula can be used through the same paracentesis to sweep posterior to the internal lip of the incision to reposit the iris (Figure 19-1). Additional help in repositing the iris may be gained by using a dispersive viscoelastic through the wound after releasing fluid pressure from behind the prolapsed iris through the paracentesis.

If decompression of the lens does not result in softening of the eye, it is highly likely that hydration of the vitreous occurred during hydrodissection. This can occur if there is some loss of zonular integrity or if the capsule has in some way been compromised with injection of the fluid directly into the vitreous space. In many cases, you can patch the eye and have the patient wait in the holding area for a few hours and the problem will resolve. In more difficult cases in which the iris prolapse cannot be controlled, you may need to proceed with a limited vitrectomy. I prefer a 25-gauge transscleral vitrectomy through a sutureless incision that is less than 1-mm, 3.5 to 4.0 mm posterior to the limbus or the use of a sharp needle on a 2-cc syringe through the sclera in the same location to draw off a few tenths of a milliliter of vitreous fluid at a time. The transscleral vitrector must be used with caution because the eye can become inordinately softened very quickly. Continuous, tactile tamponade of the globe as the vitrector is being used to monitor intraocular pressure should help avoid over-softening of the eye. Once the eye is softened adequately, further attempts at hydrodissection should not be made. Hydrodelineation can be done with less than 0.2 mL of fluid with depression of the posterior lip of the incision in order to allow egress of viscoelastic and fluid. The endonucleus should be rotatable within the epinucleus and removed, after which the epinucleus and cortex can be removed without further risk to the eye.

References

1. Fine IH. Cortical cleaving hydrodissection technique includes cortical cleanup. *Ocular Surgery News.* 1991;9:24,26-27.

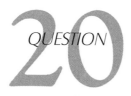
How Do I Proceed if I See a Small Wound Burn With Whitening of Corneal Stroma? How Would I Close a Severe Corneal Burn?

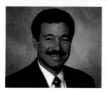

Robert H. Osher, MD

Thermal injuries during phacoemulsification range from a subtle shrinkage of collagen to a dramatic gape of a whitened incision. The former is far more common than appreciated and may appear as a thin curvilinear lucency in the incisional tunnel representing contraction of collagen where a focal thermal event has occurred. For example, if the sleeve surrounding the phaco needle is compressed against any part of the tunnel, there may be focal interruption of irrigation and increased friction between the needle and the sleeve. This can cause the temperature to rise high enough to cause the adjacent collagen to contract. Clinically, this is evident as a "shark fin" sign noted as the examiner sweeps a thin slit beam across the incision, observing a subtle curvilinear lucency.[1]

At the other end of the clinical spectrum, complete interruption of either aspiration flow or infusion can cause a rapid and sustained rise in the temperature of the phaco needle. Within seconds, transparency of the adjacent cornea is lost and the surrounding tissue whitens and coagulates, causing the lips of the incision to gape. The incision can no longer self-seal and frank leakage with inability to maintain the chamber occurs. In severe burns, the iris and cornea can be irreparably damaged.[2] What can be done to prevent this serious complication from occurring, and how can the case be salvaged should the surgeon encounter an unexpected thermal injury?

All ultrasound needles create heat by producing friction within the incision. To cool the tip of the vibrating needle, fluid bathes the barrel from the inside (aspiration flow rate) and from the outside (irrigation or infusion). There is also a minor component of fluid leakage around the tip escaping through the incision. The aspiration flow rate is the dominant variable and can be interrupted by obstructing flow with an ophthalmic viscosurgical device (OVD) or by lens material. The more retentive the OVD, the more likely it is to obstruct the aspiration flow rate so the surgeon must use enough vacuum to immediately clear a viscoelastic blockage when beginning the emulsification. Moreover, when the aspiration rate is blocked, infusion will cease so there is "double trouble" at the tip. Because I tend to use highly retentive Healon 5 (Advanced Medical Optics, Santa Ana, Calif), I must embed the ultrasound tip directly into the central anterior cortex bevel down at an initial level of 250 mm Hg, high enough to remove the emulsified lens material without the risk of OVD obstruction. Once a divot is created in the lens and there is a safe space for fluid exchange, I reduce the vacuum in accord with the principles of slow motion phacoemulsification in order to retain the OVD in the anterior chamber.[3]

The importance of proper incision construction cannot be overemphasized. As surgeons make smaller "watertight" incisions, which tend to extend more anteriorly into clear cornea, there is a greater risk for compressing the surrounding tubing through which the irrigation passes. Inadvertent "oar locking" or improper pivoting of the handpiece may kink the tubing, interrupting infusion as heat is transferred through the sleeve directly to the cornea. Even a partial obstruction may result in a focal temperature rise within the incision. Moreover, leakage may also be reduced in these tight incisions so irrigation can only occur during aspiration. If the tip becomes occluded, both irrigation and aspiration are restricted and the temperature rises. Irrigating choppers have also reduced infusion rates, and the lower pressure head may not easily move a chamber full of OVD while a sleeveless ultrasound needle is vibrating in a second incision.

During the last several years, manufacturers have added important thermal protective safeguards. All contemporary machines allow the surgeon to modulate ultrasound energy. Because friction is the dominant variable for generating heat, continuous ultrasound is the least safe option. Delivering pulses or bursts of ultrasound energy can reduce total energy. Increasing off time by lowering duty cycle is another extremely effective method in reducing heat within the incision. This innovation was introduced by the WhiteStar technology (Advanced Medical Optics). A dramatic reduction in friction and temperature has been measured with the newest Alcon technology of torsional ultrasound (Fort Worth, Tex). Different tips have been designed to maintain some flow, including the Mackool tip (Alcon, Fort Worth, Tex), which has a rigid outer sleeve, and the Barrett tip (Bausch & Lomb, Rochester, NY) with a series of longitudinal grooves that ensure infusion even if the sleeve is compressed. The ABS tip (Alcon) allows fluid to bypass an obstruction until the rising vacuum can clear the occlusion. Audible tones can warn the surgeon when occlusion occurs or when the amount of the fluid in the bottle is low.

Our laboratory studies evaluated the impact of different parameters contributing to incisional temperatures.[4] Power, duty cycle, aspiration rate, viscoelastic, vacuum, and incision size-to-tip ratio have major thermal effects. Pulse frequency, cooling the balanced salt solution (BSS), or raising the bottle height had minimal effect. A subsequent study demonstrated a thermoprotective benefit of using a coaxial set-up with ultrasleeve to allow a further reduction in incision size to 2.2 mm.[5]

The universal warning sign of thermal injury is the appearance of visible lens particles (lens milk), which represent the stagnant emulsion going nowhere. The surgeon may also

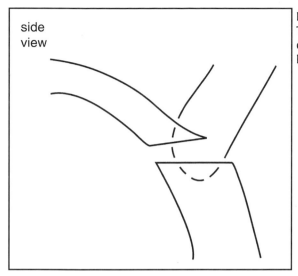

side
view

Figure 20-1. Radial "gape" suture technique. The needle passes through the proximal lip of the incision, then catches a bite of floor before exiting within the gape.

notice the lack of cutting activity or lens movement when the tip is obstructed. The surgeon must immediately abort the emulsification by decelerating the foot pedal into irrigation and aspiration (I&A) or irrigation mode in order to avoid a rapid temperature rise. Warning beeps or audible tones will alert the surgeon to an interruption of flow that can be verified by the nurse who quickly confirms the absence of activity in the drip chamber. While the surgeon may feel a temperature rise in the handpiece itself, the damage occurs in several seconds and is usually done by this point.

What Do You Do if Your Patient Has an Incisional Burn?

If the thermal injury is minimal, you may be able to complete the procedure without much fanfare. Hydration will probably fail to produce a watertight incision, in which case suture closure will likely be necessary. If the injury is more severe and a gape is present, an air bubble or an OVD may be required to prevent chamber collapse while suturing the incision is attempted. Unfortunately, a standard closure is ineffective because the incision lips are separated as if tissue has been lost. Standard suturing techniques may result in a leaking wound with extreme astigmatism.

We have developed 2 suturing options, a radial and a horizontal "gape stitch," for this purpose. The radial suture begins with the needle entering the proximal lip of the incision, then catching a bite of the floor before exiting without passing through the distal lip (Figure 20-1).[6] This method simply approximates the anterior portion of the incision, permitting a watertight closure.

The horizontal gape stitch is a trapezoidal mattress suture that begins by passing the needle of a 10-0 nylon suture radially through the posterior roof and then exiting within the incisional tunnel (Figure 20-2).[7] The needle is reloaded and passed parallel to the incision through the anterior floor, exiting within the tunnel. This needle is reloaded a third time, passing a radial bite from within the tunnel up through the posterior roof.

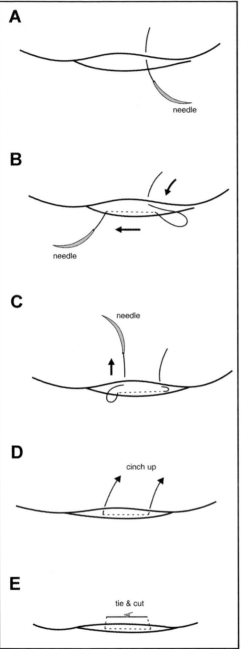

Figure 20-2. Trapezoidal "gape" suture. (A) First pass—the needle enters radially through the roof, exiting within the incisional bed. (B) Second pass—the needle is reloaded for a tangential pass through the anterior floor of the bed. Both the entry and exit sites are just lateral to the radial meridian in order to create trapezoidal configuration. (C) Third pass—the needle is reloaded, entering the tunnel to penetrate and exit through the roof. (D) The free ends of the suture are cinched and tied to form a (E) trapezoidal vertical mattress suture approximating the posterior roof to the anterior floor.

The bites through the posterior roof are slightly closer together than the bites through the anterior floor, resulting in a trapezoidal configuration. The sutures are cinched and tied, bringing the anterior floor to the posterior roof and "giving back" tissue for a watertight enclosure.

Extreme cases may require a patch-graft. However, this discussion is beyond the scope of this chapter.

Conclusion

Thermal injuries are going to occur as a complication of phacoemulsification. However, we can reduce the risk by meticulous surgical technique and the knowledgeable selection of phaco parameters. Remember, if you see lens milk, stop and figure out the problem before resuming the emulsification. Should a burn occur, try to secure the incision with a gape-suturing technique.

Acknowledgment

I would like to thank Scott E. Burk, MD, PhD and James M. Osher, MS for their assistance in writing this chapter.

References

1. Osher RH. Shark fin: a new sign of thermal injury. *J Cataract Refract Surg.* 2005;31(3):640-642.
2. Sugar A, Schertzer RM. Clinical course of phacoemulsification wound burns. *J Cataract Refract Surg.* 1999;25:688-692.
3. Osher RH, Marques DM, Marques FF, Osher JM. Slow-motion phacoemulsification technique. *Techniques in Ophthalmology.* 2003;1(2):73-79.
4. Osher RH, Injev V. Thermal study of bare tips with various system parameters and incision sizes. *J Cataract Refract Surg.* 2006;32:867-872.
5. Osher RH, Injev V. Microcoaxial phacoemulsification: laboratory study. *J Cataract Refract Surg.* In press.
6. Osher RH. Gape stitch. *Video Journal of Cataract and Refractive Surgery.* 1990;VI(3).
7. Osher RH. Thermal burns. *Video Journal of Cataract and Refractive Surgery.* 1993;IX(3).

HOW SHOULD I
MANAGE A SMALL OR LARGE
DESCEMET'S MEMBRANE DETACHMENT?

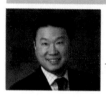

Terry Kim, MD

The incidence of Descemet's membrane (DM) detachments has been cited to be as high as 43%,[1] and cataract surgery has been reported to be a major predisposing factor.[2] Fortunately, the majority of these detachments are small, localized to the wound(s), and clinically insignificant. However, at times, these small detachments can extend during surgery to become moderate or large-sized detachments that require attention and treatment.

In cataract surgery, DM detachments usually occur at the site of the clear corneal wound and/or paracentesis incision. By far, the most common cause is a dull blade that causes a focal tear/separation of DM from the stroma (Figure 21-1). The repeated introduction of instruments and devices through these wounds (ie, the phacoemulsification tip, irrigation/aspiration [I/A] tip, viscoelastic cannula, balanced salt solution [BSS] cannula, intraocular lens [IOL] cartridge, IOL) can cause these localized tears/detachments to extend and enlarge. In particular, any blunt edge of an instrument or device (ie, the sleeve of the phaco or I/A tip, the tip of the IOL cartridge, the edge of the IOL) can "catch" the edge of DM during entry into the clear corneal wound and further strip the membrane (Figure 21-2). Forceful insertion of a viscoelastic/BSS cannula tip or second instrument (ie, Koch nucleus spatula, Kuglen hook [Katena Products Inc, Denville, NJ]) through the paracentesis incision can also cause DM to tear and detach. The injection of BSS or viscoelastic prior to complete entry of the cannula tip into the anterior chamber can also cause severe DM detachments.

Because these detachments start in the peripheral cornea at the internal incision sites (and then extend centrally), they can be difficult to detect and visualize. After wound

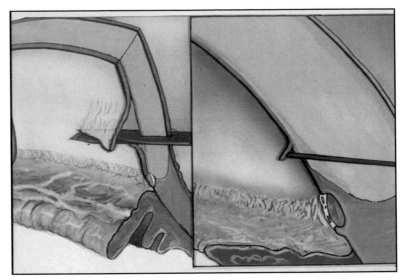

Figure 21-1. This illustration depicts how a dull blade can cause DM to tear and separate from the corneal stroma. (From Fishkind WJ, ed. *Complications in Phacoemulsification: Avoidance, Recognition, and Management.* New York, NY: Thieme Medical Publishers; 2002. Reprinted with permission.)

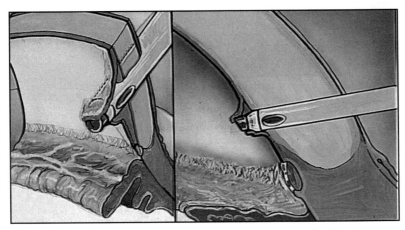

Figure 21-2. This diagram demonstrates how small DM tears or detachments can enlarge or extend upon insertion of an instrument through the corneal incision. (From Fishkind WJ, ed. *Complications in Phacoemulsification: Avoidance, Recognition, and Management.* New York, NY: Thieme Medical Publishers; 2002. Reprinted with permission.)

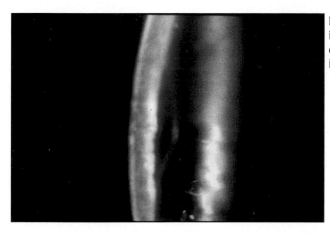

Figure 21-3. Slit-lamp photograph illustrating a paracentral, localized DM detachment with no evidence of tearing or scrolling.

construction, the surgeon is typically focused on the central aspects of the cornea/anterior chamber/lens during the cataract extraction. Furthermore, common conditions like arcus senilis and stromal hydration/edema of the corneal wounds prohibit good visualization of the posterior layers of the peripheral cornea. When these defects in DM are noted intraoperatively, they are recognized incidentally as a torn edge or scroll of DM during instrument/device insertion, or if more extensive, as a frank DM detachment flapping in the anterior chamber during cataract surgery (Figure 21-3).

Prevention

Routine steps can be taken during cataract surgery to help prevent tears or detachments of DM:

* First, a sharp blade—whether it is metal or diamond—should be used for all incisions. If any substantial resistance during wound construction is encountered, the blade should be removed, inspected, and preferably replaced with a new blade.

* Avoid forceful insertion of any instrument/device by altering the angle of insertion and/or enlarging the clear cornea and/or paracentesis incision.

* When injecting viscoelastic or other substances into the anterior chamber, the surgeon should always ensure that the cannula tip has passed completely through the cornea into the anterior chamber before initiating the injection to prevent dissection of DM from the stroma.

Once a DM tear or detachment is noted intraoperatively, certain precautions should be taken to avoid further damage to DM, particularly the anterior portion that lies superior to the incision site because of its potential to extend centrally:

* Special attention should be given to posterior corneal abnormalities, particularly Fuchs' endothelial dystrophy. These conditions probably predispose the patient to easier stripping of DM during cataract surgery due to a compromised endothelial pump.

* Careful visualization of instruments/devices under higher magnification during insertion can help to prevent "catching" DM.

∗ Because it is more crucial to avoid the anterior portion of DM, placing more posterior pressure on the posterior lip of the incision during instrument/device insertion can help avoid further stripping of DM centrally.

∗ Enlarging the incision and lubricating the incision with viscoelastic can ease the entry of instrument/device insertion through a tight wound.

∗ A dispersive (Viscoat, Alcon, Fort Worth, Tex) or adaptive (Healon 5, Advanced Medical Optics, Santa Ana, Calif) viscoelastic can also be used to provide a temporary tamponade of the detachment. An alternate incision site is recommended (ie, the paracentesis incision is used for viscoelastic tamponade of DM detachment at the clear corneal incision and vice versa), and extra precaution needs to be taken to ensure that viscoelastic is NOT injected between the DM and the stroma.

Treatment

For small DM detachments noted intraoperatively, no particular treatment is generally necessary. However, moderate or large-sized detachments may necessitate aborting the cataract procedure and warrant intraoperative treatment with either air or gas tamponade or perhaps suturing at the conclusion of the case. The DM tear or scroll may need to be repositioned prior to tamponade treatment, and if so, excessive manipulation and direct contact with DM with any instrument should be avoided to minimize endothelial loss (if the detached DM is too torn, shredded, or scrolled, air/gas injection alone will not suffice). Intracameral air injection lasts shorter than gas and should be used for smaller detachments. For more extensive DM detachments, I recommend the injection of a non-expansive 20% concentration of sulfur hexafluoride (SF6) gas with approximately 60% to 70% fill of the anterior chamber (Figure 21-4). With either air or gas injection, proper head positioning may be required to ensure that the bubble is positioned correctly against the DM. These patients should be followed closely for intraocular pressure monitoring and DM reattachment and should be given cycloplegic medications to avoid pupillary block glaucoma.

Frequently, DM detachments are not noted until slit-lamp examination is performed postoperatively. Clinically, these patients can present with severe corneal edema overlying the DM detachment that can make the diagnosis difficult. The use of topical glycerin to temporarily clear the edema or imaging modalities (ie, anterior segment optical coherence tomography or ultrasound biomicroscopy) can help confirm the diagnosis (Figure 21-5). Topical corticosteroid therapy and observation are usually the first steps of treatment with the hopes of spontaneous DM reattachment. For persistent DM detachments, the same aforementioned techniques utilizing air or gas can be used to reattach DM. Of note, we published a new, simplified technique for reattaching DM detachments postoperatively using intracameral 20% SF6 gas that can be performed with minimal instruments in a minor operating room or at the slit-lamp microscope.[3] Finally, various transcorneal suturing techniques may be necessary to address the more severe and refractory DM detachments.[4]

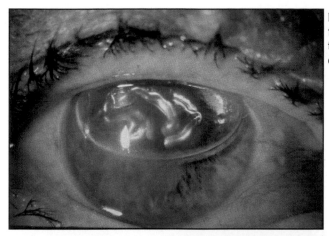

Figure 21-4. A 20% SF6 gas bubble fills 60% of the anterior chamber to tamponade a large, central DM detachment.

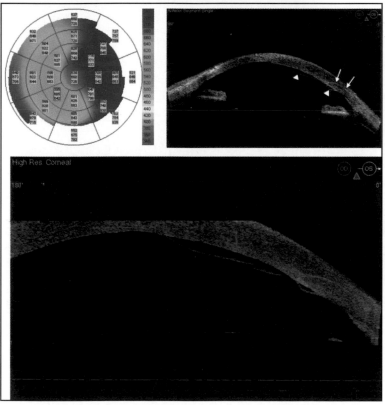

Figure 21-5. Anterior segment OCT of Descemet's membrane detachment after cataract surgery. (The orientation of these scans is nasal to temporal going from left to right.) The pachymetric map in the upper left shows sectoral edema temporally as indicated by the cooler, darker blues. The view of the anterior segment in the upper right corner shows the temporal clear corneal wound (arrows) and Descemet's membrane detached from the cornea proper (arrowheads). The bottom image provides a higher resolution view.

Prognosis

The prognosis for small to moderate DM detachments remains excellent, especially with the more recently described technique of intracameral gas injection. However, permanent corneal decompensation can ensue with severe detachments and require corneal transplantation. In this scenario, a posterior lamellar approach (ie, Descemet's stripping endothelial keratoplasty or DSEK) can help minimize incision size, reduce postoperative astigmatism, and hasten visual recovery. In general, the surprising resiliency of the corneal endothelium allows these cells to remain viable even in the state of DM detachment so that continued pump function can resume upon successful treatment.

References

1. Monroe WD. Gonioscopy after cataract extraction. *South Med J.* 1971;64:1122.
2. Pieramici D, Green WR, Stark WJ. Stripping of Descemet's membrane: a clinicopathologic correlation. *Ophthalmic Surg.* 1994;25(4):226-231.
3. Kim T, Hasan SA. A new technique for repairing Descemet membrane detachments using intracameral gas injection. *Arch Ophthalmol.* 2002;120(2):181-183.
4. Olson RJ. Corneal problems associated with phacoemulsification. In: Fishkind WJ, ed. *Complications in Phacoemulsification: Recognition, Avoidance, and Management.* New York, NY: Thieme Medical Publishing; 2002.

AFTER INSERTING THE PHACO TIP, THE CHAMBER DRAMATICALLY DEEPENS AND THE PATIENT COMPLAINS OF PAIN. HOW SHOULD I PROCEED?

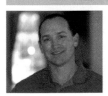

Robert J. Cionni, MD

Cataract surgery in the highly myopic eye presents several challenges. Intraocular lens (IOL) calculation is more difficult and with a less certain outcome. A higher risk of retinal detachment exists. Additionally, the surgical procedure itself may be more complex to perform and more uncomfortable for the patient due to the higher possibility of lens-iris diaphragm retropulsion syndrome (LIDRS).

In 1995, Hans Wilbrandt, MD described, characterized, and discussed the etiology and management of LIDRS.[1] He noted that upon instigating infusion into the anterior chamber during phacoemulsification or automated cortical aspiration, the pupil would dilate widely, the peripheral iris would bow posteriorly, and the anterior chamber would deepen dramatically (Figure 22-1). He postulated that this syndrome was more common in the myopic patient whose need to accommodate for near vision was less. Therefore, the ciliary muscles and zonules never become strong or taut. Thus, when hydrostatic pressure is induced anterior to the iris, posterior bowing and movement can occur more easily than in an eye with taut zonules and strong ciliary muscles. Dr. Wilbrandt suggested lowering the height of the infusion bottle to decrease the anterior chamber pressure. Since this would simultaneously induce anterior chamber volatility, he also advocated a second infusion line with the bottle height also low. Despite these efforts, phacoemulsification in these eyes remained difficult with a significant degree of chamber volatility.

Figure 22-1. LIDRS. The pupil dilates widely, the peripheral iris bows posteriorly, and the chamber deepens dramatically.

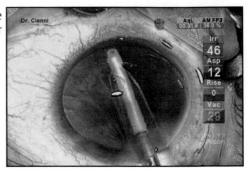

The evolution of small incision phacoemulsification within a closed system and ever-rising bottle heights has accentuated the incidence and significance of LIDRS. The anterior chamber pressure induced by a high infusion bottle combined with nonleaking incisions can be quite significant. Additionally, as many surgeons who have moved to topical anesthesia have discovered, LIDRS is quite uncomfortable for the patient. So what can we do to manage LIDRS so that the procedure can become more routine for the surgeon and more comfortable for the patient?

In order to effectively manage LIDRS, we need to better understand its etiology. As surgeons began the move to smaller incisions for phacoemulsification, we also began to utilize continuous circular capsulorrhexis (CCC), a surgical technique that seems to encourage LIDRS. With a continuous anterior capsular rim upon which the iris can "seal," a reverse pupillary block (RPB) can occur. Once the anterior segment is sealed from the posterior segment, any anterior pressure can push the iris-capsular bag complex posteriorly. If one watches carefully, insignificant RPB occurs in almost every case of phacoemulsification. However, full-blown LIDRS is prevented in most by a strong ciliozonular apparatus and a well-formed vitreous. In those individuals who have a weakened ciliozonular apparatus or who have had previous vitrectomy, the RPB allows the ciliary body to stretch and bow posteriorly, bringing with it the peripheral iris. The higher the bottle, the more significant the deepening will become.

If it is necessary for a RPB to occur in order to induce LIDRS, then disrupting the RPB should resolve LIDRS. Indeed, by simply lifting the iris off of the residual anterior capsular rim, the chamber depth does normalize, the peripheral iris flattens, the pupil returns to normal size, and the patient's sensation of painful pressure is alleviated (Figure 22-2).[2] Typically, the resolution is immediate but with use of a higher viscosity viscoelastic agent, the iris may need to be lifted for nearly 360 degrees before this maneuver is successful. Additionally, each time a new irrigating instrument is introduced, LIDRS will likely reoccur. One can place a dull instrument under the iris to maintain a space before beginning infusion to prevent the onset of LIDRS. Alternatively, as suggested by Lisa B. Arbisser, MD, place a small amount of viscoelastic between the iris and anterior capsule to maintain this space and prevent RPB. Either technique may prevent LIDRS from occurring.

Surgery in the highly myopic eye has posed several challenges, including LIDRS. Understanding that RPB leads to LIDRS now allows us to more effectively manage these eyes. Reversal of RPB is accomplished with a simple maneuver that results in quick resolution of LIDRS and thereby provides these patients with a more comfortable and safer procedure.

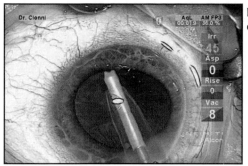

Figure 22-2. Separating the iris from the anterior capsule resolves the LIDRS.

References

1. Wilbrandt HR, Wilbrandt TH. Pathogenesis and management of the lens-iris diaphragm retropulsion syndrome during phacoemulsification. *J Cataract Refract Surg.* 1994;20:48-53.
2. Cionni R, Osher R, Barros M. Management of lens-iris diaphragm retropulsion syndrome during phacoemulsification. *J Cataract Refract Surg.* 2004;30(5):953-956.

WHAT SHOULD I DO DIFFERENTLY WITH A POSTERIOR POLAR CATARACT?

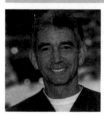

Samuel F. Masket, MD

Posterior polar cataract represents one of the uniquely challenging situations for the anterior segment surgeon. The condition, a dominantly inherited disorder with variable expressivity, may be associated with intraoperative defects in the posterior capsule. Because the condition is dominantly inherited, typically both eyes are involved and there is no gender preference. However, posterior lenticonus, a similar physical phenomenon, is more typically uniocular, has a tendency for females, and is generally diagnosed in the first decade of life. Previous publications indicate as high as a 26% likelihood for a defective capsule at the time of cataract surgery.[1] It is unclear whether the defect in the capsule is pre-existent or develops iatrogenically because of marked thinning.

Can one tell if the capsule is defective prior to surgery? Daljit Singh, an extraordinarily prolific Indian surgeon, has described a sign that he suggests is indicative of a defect in the capsule. His sign is that of a series of satellite minicataracts surrounding the main posterior polar plaque. In his view, the congenitally defective capsule allows aqueous to permeate into the lens material and induce small secondary opacities. In my surgical experience, a defective capsule in one eye is most often met with a defective capsule in the second eye. Likewise, the earlier in life the patient presents with symptoms, the greater the likelihood for a defective capsule. Conversely, elderly patients with posterior polar cataract in addition to nuclear or other age-related cataract formation, in my experience, tend not to have defective capsules.

Most patients with posterior polar cataracts present with symptoms as they start to become presbyopic because the loss of accommodation teams with the evolving cataract near the nodal point to significantly reduce reading ability. Physical findings most

Figure 23-1. Classic appearance of central posterior polar cataract.

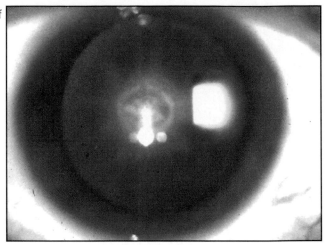

typically are that of a fully normal examination with the exception of the posterior polar plaque-like cataract, which is three-dimensional; it may have the appearance of a hockey puck (Figure 23-1). I have not been impressed with any other typical abnormalities in eyes with posterior polar cataracts.

In any case, because of the proclivity for a defective posterior capsule in a significant proportion of cases, a surgical strategy must be adapted in order to preclude serious intraoperative complications should capsule rupture occur. Moreover, the strategy will prepare the surgeon for dealing with capsule rupture under other circumstances. When counseling such a patient in preparation for surgery, I spend considerable time discussing the increased risk and nature of complications. I may spend as much chair time discussing the situation as I do operative time fixing the problem.

Experienced surgeons should be comfortable with topical/intracameral anesthesia; however, given the likelihood for prolonged surgery, one might plan for alternative anesthetic strategies and be prepared to convert to sub-Tenon's infiltration intraoperatively.

Incisional and astigmatism considerations are routine; however, one should be certain to create a self-sealing incision in order to avoid shallowing of the anterior chamber as instruments are removed. The anterior capsulorrhexis is of particular importance. If the posterior capsule is defective, it is very beneficial to use the remaining anterior capsule to capture the optic of the implant (Figure 23-2). Therefore, the capsulorrhexis must be intact, well centered, and somewhat smaller than the size of the planned optic. With respect to machine fluidic parameters, given a risk for a defect in the posterior capsule it is wise to reduce inflow during surgery. As a result, aspiration flow rate and vacuum must also be lowered, in keeping with the "slow motion" technique described by Osher.[1]

The surgical hallmark in management of posterior polar cataract is avoiding hydrodissection because hydrostatic pressure may "blow out" the defective or weakened posterior capsule. Instead, hydrodelineation is employed to separate the endonucleus from the epinucleus and cortex. As a rule, the endonucleus is soft and can be removed by simple emulsification without the need for rotation, which risks stressing the posterior capsule. Should the nucleus be firmer, vertical chopping and elevation of the nuclear halves away from the epinucleus is a generally successful strategy. Following removal of the endonucleus, I use a dispersive ophthalmic viscosurgical device (OVD) to dissect the cortex

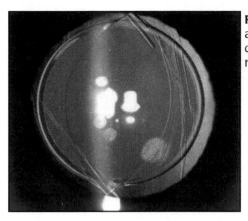

Figure 23-2. Optic capture. The IOL loops are situated anterior to the capsule bag while the optic has been deliberately displaced behind the anterior capsulorrhexis, creating stable fixation.

and epinucleus away from the posterior capsule. Generally, I employ small aliquots in multiple locations but do not allow the agent to reach the posterior pole of the lens. Next, I use bimanual irrigation and aspiration (I/A) (this affords a safety factor if the capsule opens) to remove the cortex and epinucleus from the peripheral aspect of the capsule bag, leaving behind the posterior polar plaque until all other lens material has been aspirated. In this manner, should the capsule rent, little to no material can fall into the posterior segment. If the capsule remains intact, surgery is routine from this point forward. However, the capsule will often have small fragments of residual lens opacity. I prefer to leave these and open the capsule with the Nd:YAG laser postoperatively as necessary.

On the other hand, if a rent in the capsule occurs, the surgeon should not withdraw the handpieces rapidly from the eye. Instead, the infusion bottle should be lowered, only the aspiration device removed, and air or OVD added to maintain a formed anterior chamber as the infusing handpiece is removed. Hopefully, that strategy will prevent anterior movement of the vitreous and extension of the capsular defect; in turn, this may allow the surgeon to convert the defect into a posterior circular capsulorrhexis. Nonetheless, in my experience, once the capsule ruptures, the defect extends rapidly because the capsule is thinner than normal. In the presence of a capsule defect, I remove all remaining cortex with a low flow or "dry" bimanual fashion; residual cortex, especially when mixed with vitreous, can induce long-term inflammation and cystoid macular edema. It is also essential to remove vitreous from the anterior chamber bimanually; this may be facilitated by a pars plana approach and with the use of triamcinolone staining of the vitreous. Once the anterior segment is free of cortex and vitreous, an intraocular lens may be implanted as dictated by the condition of the anterior/posterior capsules. As mentioned above, it is my preference to place the IOL in the ciliary sulcus and then capture the optic behind the anterior capsule. The viscoagent is removed bimanually either with I/A or with the automated vitrector. As with all cataract surgery, I leave the eye at physiologic intraocular pressure and test all incisions with fluorescein dye to assure hermetic sealing.

References

1. Osher RH, Yu BC, Koch DD. Posterior polar cataracts: a predisposition to intraoperative posterior capsular rupture. *J Cataract Refract Surg.* 1990;16(2):157-162.

WHAT SHOULD I DO DIFFERENTLY WITH A HYPERMATURE WHITE CATARACT?

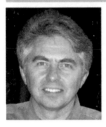

Steve A. Arshinoff, MD, FRCSC

Whenever I see a new patient with unilateral or bilateral hypermature white cataracts, I ask myself, "Why is this patient presenting so late?" It is a crucial question to ask yourself if you want to assure successful treatment. The first step in management is a very careful history. Is the cataract traumatic, perhaps hiding some occult broken zonules? Is the patient a recent immigrant who speaks no English? Is he or she an alcoholic, brought in by a relative, and likely to have been subject to repeated ocular trauma? Is there a past unadmitted history of ocular disease, and the patient is presenting to "the great doctor" for a miracle cure? No possibility can be excluded without investigation in these patients because factors such as these can affect management and outcome.

Preoperative Management

The first step in managing these patients is a careful preoperative assessment. A relative afferent papillary defect will tell you that something, other than the cataract, is wrong with this eye. A fully dilated exam will expose things like broken zonules, phacodonesis, a crenated surface of the cataract, an unusually deep or shallow anterior chamber (AC), some idea of the nuclear density behind the white cortex, and perhaps even a peek at the retina through some relatively clear area of the lens. If the retina cannot be examined, a B scan should be done at the same time as biometry of both eyes, and if possible, an IOLMaster (Carl Zeiss Meditec, Jena, Germany) assessment of the contralateral eye. You want to know if there is significant anisometropia and perhaps amblyopia. Bilateral

Figure 24-1. Painting Vision*Blue* over the anterior capsule. (Reprinted from *J Cataract Refract Surg, 31,* Arshinoff SA. Letter. Capsular dyes and the USST, 259-260, © 2005, with permission from ASCRS & ESCRS.)

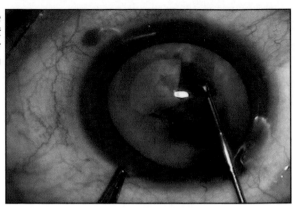

corneal topography may demonstrate asymmetrical astigmatism, again suggesting that amblyopia may be the reason the cataract was left to mature. I always warn these patients that they may have some pathology that I have not discovered, despite the investigations, and that the surgical prognosis must remain guarded until I can do a complete examination postoperatively.

Surgery

The difficult part of operating on hypermature cataracts occurs right at the beginning of surgery. Performing a continuous circular capsulorrhexis (CCC) in such cases with an inadequately pressurized eye often results in the "Argentinean flag syndrome." This is due to the tendency of the capsulorrhexis to tear outward to the equator as soon as the trypan blue-stained capsule is punctured if the pressure behind the lens is not equalized with anterior pressure from an elastic ophthalmic viscosurgical device (OVD) (ie, high viscosity and cohesive). So I do the following:

* A <1-mm side-port incision is made (incisional leakage allows the eye to depressurize and encourages the Argentinean flag syndrome), through which I inject 1% non-preserved, isotonic lidocaine. This provides excellent anesthesia, maintains intraocular pressure, and further dilates the pupil if left in for 1 minute or more.

* The primary incision is made tight and a bit longer into the cornea than usual, again to assure against leakage.

* The AC is filled about 90% with Healon 5 (Advanced Medical Optics, Santa Ana, Calif) (or other viscoadaptive). The very high viscosity and cohesion of viscoadaptives permit the chamber to be filled until the center of the lens capsule is seen to indent, indicating that a "pressure-equalized" state has been reached.

* I then paint trypan blue over the capsular surface, below the Healon 5 layer in the Ultimate Soft Shell-Trypan Blue Technique (Figure 24-1).[1] Since the early 1990s, many agents have been tried for capsular staining. Indocyanine green (ICG) was found to be toxic and yielded inferior visibility compared to trypan blue. Trypan blue, prepared commercially and sold as Vision*Blue* by the Dutch Ophthalmic Research Corporation (DORC) (Rotterdam, Holland), has proved to yield the best

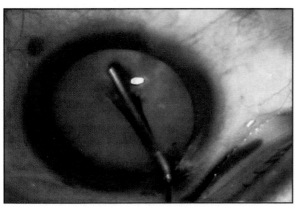

Figure 24-2. USST modified for trypan blue. Note extremely clear view. (Reprinted from *J Cataract Refract Surg, 31,* Arshinoff SA. Letter. Capsular dyes and the USST, 259-260, © 2005, with permission from ASCRS & ESCRS.)

visibility, have the least toxicity, and further assist by decreasing capsular elasticity in a time-dependent fashion over 1 minute. (This makes it excellent for pediatric cataracts surgery.) After painting a single drop of trypan blue over the capsule under the viscoadaptive layer, I then irrigate any excess gently with a small amount of intracameral xylocaine, and fully pressurize the eye in the ultimate soft shell technique (USST) style.[1] The capsulorrhexis is then fashioned with a 27-gauge needle that I bend myself, keeping it at about 5 mm in diameter, further assuring that I do not cause Argentinean flag syndrome (Figure 24-2). This technique yields an extremely clear view of the capsule. If areas of fibrosis or calcification are present in the anterior capsule, the capsulorrhexis can be done with diathermy or a curved Vannas scissors, simply going around these areas where possible. Resorting to a can-opener technique is to be discouraged.

⁎ Hydrodissection is easy with a hypermature white cataract but should not be omitted. It is important to get as much white cortex out of the way as possible, before beginning phaco, because it will obscure the surgical view. Small bursts of fluid injected under the capsulorrhexis edge in about 4 positions around the clock will usually suffice to free up most of the white cortex. When the phaco is first inserted into the eye, the inside edge of the capsulorrhexis should be encircled under aspiration or very low phaco power in order to aspirate as much remaining cortex as possible before approaching the nucleus.

⁎ Finally, we get to the nucleus. At this point, a careful assessment of the apparent lens density is appropriate. It can be anything from a soft, seminecrotic blob to a black 4+ rock. But it is usually free floating in the capsular bag, which makes all sculpting techniques inadvisable. My preference is to use my own variant of vertical chopping, called "phaco slice and separate."[2] Briefly, the nucleus is impaled with the phaco tip to stabilize it, and it is then sliced with a Nagahara chopper or Shepherd tomahawk. I call it "slice" because if the nucleus is very dense, it can be repeatedly sliced until cleavage is obtained, somewhat like slicing bread. It is not always possible to "chop" very dense or very soft lenses, but all can be sliced. I prefer to use the Alcon Infiniti machine (Fort Worth, Tex) with coaxial Custom Ozil settings and intermittent continuously variable axial and torsional pulse, but linear pulse works well on most machines. The phaco should be done with care because there is no cortical shell present for capsular protection. It is preferable to slice all the nuclear pieces x 360 degrees before beginning removal in these dense lenses. The unremoved sliced-off nuclear fragments stabilize the capsular bag while further slicing is completed. The remainder of the procedure is pretty standard once the nucleus is removed.

Conclusion

The most challenging part of operating on hypermature white cataracts is the capsulorrhexis. Preventing loss of pressurization of the AC, use of Vision*Blue*, and observing a few of the precautions I have mentioned should make your future dealings with these cases almost routine, and very satisfying.

References

1. Arshinoff SA. Letter. Capsular dyes and the USST. *J Cataract Refract Surg.* 2005;31:259-260.
2. Arshinoff SA. Phaco slice and separate. *J Cataract Refract Surg.* 1999;25(4):474-478.

WHAT IS THE BEST WAY TO MANAGE INTRAOPERATIVE FLOPPY IRIS SYNDROME?

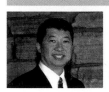

David F. Chang, MD

Intraoperative floppy iris syndrome (IFIS) is most commonly associated with tamsulosin (Flomax, Boehringer Ingelheim Pharmaceuticals, Inc, Ridgefield, Conn). A triad of intraoperative signs—iris billowing and floppiness, iris prolapse to the main and side incisions, and progressive miosis—characterize IFIS (Figure 25-1).[1] While other systemic alpha-1 blockers such as doxazosin (Cardura, Pfizer, Inc, New York, NY), terazosin (Hytrin, Abbott, Chicago, Ill), and alfuzosin (Uroxatral, sanofi-aventis, Bridgewater, NJ) can also cause IFIS, the frequency and severity of IFIS is much less when compared with tamsulosin. This difference probably reflects the stronger affinity and specificity of tamsulosin for the alpha-1A receptor subtype that predominates in both the prostate and the iris dilator muscle.[2,3]

Because there is significant variability in IFIS severity between different patients, and even between both eyes of the same patient, it is difficult to conclude whether one management technique is superior to another. In fact, the varied IFIS strategies discussed below are often complementary and surgeons should gain experience with several approaches. We can categorize IFIS as being mild (good dilation; some iris billowing without prolapse or constriction), moderate (iris billowing without prolapse, but with constriction of a moderately dilated pupil), or severe (classic triad and poor preoperative dilation). In one prospective study of 167 eyes in patients taking tamsulosin, the distribution of IFIS severity using this scale was as follows: 10% no IFIS, 17% mild, 30% moderate, and 43% severe.[3]

Several adjunctive pharmacologic approaches to managing IFIS have been proposed.[2,4] Stopping tamsulosin preoperatively is of unpredictable and questionable value as there

Figure 25-1. Iris billowing, prolapse to phaco and side-port incision, and pupil constriction in a patient taking tamsulosin.

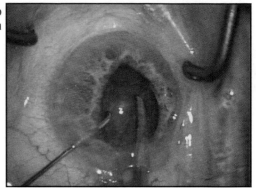

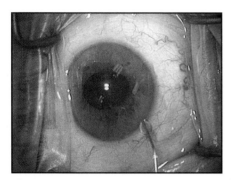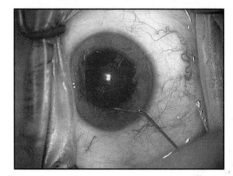

Figure 25-2. Intracameral epinephrine (1:1000 bisulfite-free, mixed 1:3 with BSS) injected in eye of patient on tamsulosin.

are many documented cases of IFIS occurring up to several years following drug cessation. Preoperative atropine drops (eg, 1% 3 times a day for 1 day to 2 days preoperatively) will maximize cycloplegia. However, this strategy alone is often ineffective for moderate to severe IFIS. If preoperative atropine is used, stopping tamsulosin could cause acute urinary retention. Direct intracameral injection of alpha agonists such as phenylephrine and epinephrine can further dilate the pupil and restore iris rigidity by increasing iris dilator smooth muscle tone (Figure 25-2).[4] Even if the pupil does not dilate further, these agents may prevent iris billowing and prolapse. One should avoid preserved solutions and use a diluted mixture (eg, 1:1000 bisulfite-free epinephrine [American Regent] mixed 1:3 with balanced salt solution [BSS] or BSS+) in order to buffer the pH.

As for general surgical principles, be attentive to proper incision construction, perform hydrodissection more gently and slowly than usual, and use lower irrigation and aspiration flow parameters if possible. Partial thickness sphincterotomies and mechanical pupil stretching are ineffective for IFIS and may exacerbate the prolapse and miosis. Bimanual microincisional cataract surgery may be helpful, particularly for mild to moderate IFIS. In addition to permitting tighter incisions, the irrigation currents can be more easily isolated within the anterior chamber, resulting in less billowing and prolapse of the iris.

Of all the ophthalmic viscosurgical devices, Healon 5 (Advanced Medical Optics. Santa Ana, Calif) has particular utility in these cases.[5] Its maximally cohesive properties are ideal for viscomydriasis and for blocking iris prolapse. Unlike classic cohesive agents, however, Healon 5 will not be immediately evacuated at lower flow and vacuum rates (eg, <175 mm Hg to 200 mm Hg; <26 mL/min). As Healon 5 is aspirated, supplemental

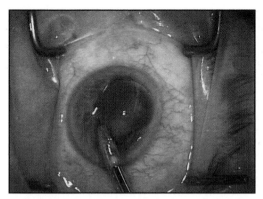 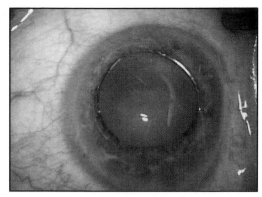

Figure 25-3. Morcher 5S PMMA pupil expansion ring inserted with the injector in an IFIS patient.

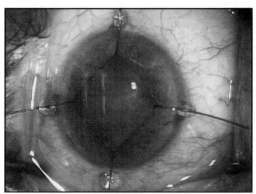

Figure 25-4. Reusable 4-0 Prolene iris retractors placed in a diamond configuration. The subincisional hook is through a separate stab incision made just posterior to and beneath the temporal clear corneal incision.

reinjections become necessary. This strategy is less suitable if high vacuum settings are desired for denser nuclei. Injecting Healon 5 peripherally over the iris and then filling the central chamber with a dispersive agent, such as Viscoat (Alcon, Fort Worth, Tex), creates a Healon 5 "donut." The latter will better resist aspiration and delay the evacuation of Healon 5.

Disposable pupil expansion rings are costly but 100% effective. Both the Morcher 5S Pupil Ring (Morcher GmbH, Stuttgart, Germany) and the Milvella PerfectPupil (Milvella Limited, Epping, Australia) are grooved polymethylmethacrylate (PMMA) rings that are threaded alongside the pupillary margin using metal injectors (Figure 25-3). A disposable plastic injector is used to insert Eagle Vision's Graether silicone pupil expansion ring (Memphis, Tenn). All of these rings are more difficult to position if the pupil is less than 4 mm wide or if the anterior chamber is shallow.

Iris retractors are another 100% reliable strategy for pupil expansion with IFIS. One-mm limbal paracenteses are made in each quadrant, including a separate stab incision made just posterior to the temporal clear corneal incision. Placement of the hooks in this diamond configuration has several significant advantages (Figure 25-4).[6] The subincisional hook retracts the iris downward and out of the path of the phaco tip. This maximizes exposure in front of the phaco tip while the nasal hook facilitates chopper placement.

If the pupil is fibrotic, such as with chronic pilocarpine use or long-standing posterior synechiae, overstretching it with iris retractors can cause bleeding, sphincter tears, and permanent mydriasis. This usually does not occur with the IFIS pupil, which is so elastic that it readily springs back to physiologic size despite being maximally stretched. I prefer reusable 4-0 polypropylene retractors (Katena, FCI) to 6-0 nylon disposable retractors (Alcon). Being of the same size and stiffness as an intraocular lens haptic, the former are more easily manipulated and can be repeatedly autoclaved, making them very cost effective to use.

It is much easier and safer to insert iris retractors and pupil expansion rings prior to capsulorrhexis initiation. If the pupil dilates very poorly or billows during injection of intracameral lidocaine, one should anticipate severe IFIS and consider using these mechanical devices. Often, however, the pupil dilates reasonably well, and it is not until after hydrodissection or during phaco that the prolapse and miosis occur. Healon 5 and intracameral epinephrine are excellent "rescue" techniques in this situation where it is difficult to see the capsulorrhexis edge. If one chooses to insert iris retractors at this point, it is useful to retract the pupil margin with a second instrument to avoid snagging the capsulorrhexis margin with the retractors.

Eliciting a history of alpha-blocker use allows surgeons to anticipate IFIS and to employ these varied strategies either alone or in combination. The previously mentioned prospective, multicenter trial using these techniques in 167 consecutive eyes from patients on tamsulosin demonstrated excellent outcomes and only a 0.6% posterior capsular rupture rate.[3]

Understanding the variability in IFIS severity associated with tamsulosin and other alpha-1 blockers and being proficient with multiple approaches allow surgeons to use a staged approach in dealing with this condition.[4] Pharmacologic measures alone are usually adequate for mild to moderate IFIS cases. Whether they expand the pupil or not, intracameral epinephrine and phenylephrine usually reduce iris billowing and prolapse by increasing iris dilator muscle tone. If the pupil diameter is still suboptimal, Healon 5 can further expand it for the capsulorrhexis or phaco. Finally, mechanical expansion devices provide reliable and optimal surgical exposure for severe IFIS and should be considered when other surgical risk factors (eg dense nuclei, weak zonules) are present.

Acknowledgments

I wish to acknowledge those who, to my knowledge, were the earliest proponents of the IFIS strategies mentioned in this chapter: Sam Masket (atropine), Richard Packard and David Allen (intracameral phenylephrine), Joel Shugar (intracameral epinephrine), Bob Osher and Doug Koch (Healon 5), Steve Arshinoff (Healon 5 "soft shell" [Viscoat peripheral + H5 central]), and Wendell Scott (Healon 5 "donut" [H5 peripheral + Viscoat central]).

References

1. Chang DF, Campbell JR. Intraoperative floppy iris syndrome associated with tamsulosin (Flomax). *J Cataract Refract Surg*. 2005;31:664-673.
2. Chang DF. Intraoperative floppy iris syndrome. In: Agarwal A, ed. *Phaco Nightmares: Conquering Cataract Catastrophes*. Thorofare, NJ: SLACK Incorporated; 2006.
3. Chang DF, Osher RH, Wang L, Koch DD. A prospective multicenter evaluation of cataract surgery in patients taking tamsulosin (Flomax). *Ophthalmology*. 2007; in press.
4. Manvikar S, Allen D. Cataract surgery management in patients taking tamsulosin. *J Cataract Refract Surg*. 2006;32:1611-1614.
5. Arshinoff SA. Modified SST-USST for tamsulosin-associated intraocular floppy iris syndrome. *J Cataract Refract Surg*. 2006;32:559-561.
6. Oetting TA, Omphroy LC. Modified technique using flexible iris retractors in clear corneal surgery. *J Cataract Refract Surg*. 2002;28:596-598.

AFTER CHOPPING OR CRACKING A 4+ NUCLEUS, A LEATHERY POSTERIOR PLATE STILL CONNECTS THE FRAGMENTS CENTRALLY. HOW SHOULD I PROCEED?

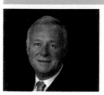

Roger F. Steinert, MD

The most challenging aspect of phacoemulsification of the 4+ nucleus is the resistance of the posterior nucleus to a clean cleavage of the cracked segments. This is true whether you are performing divide and conquer, horizontal chop, or vertical chop. To deal with the phenomenon, you have to understand its origin. By the time a cataract reaches the 4+ stage, the expansion of the nuclear hardening has incorporated the epinucleus. The posterior epinucleus is no longer a malleable separate cushion layer. Instead, it is firmer and adherent to the endonucleus. When you try to split the endonucleus, the posterior layer has bridging fibers that we have come to call "leathery." Another analogy is the "green-stick fracture" phenomenon that occurs when you try to break a fresh tree branch. The fibers do not break cleanly, but rather flex and keep the 2 ends of the branch connected.

The net result is that you can separate the nuclear fragments you create, but when you try to engage and remove the fragment with vacuum, it will only come partially and then fall back. The phenomenon of the bridging posterior strands is maximal at the center of the posterior nucleus, which means that the apex of the nuclear fragment not only remains adherent, but also cannot be tilted to be engaged by the phaco tip. The result is a stranded posterior plate (Figure 26-1A).

In theory, you might think that flipping the nucleus, so that the posterior portion is now anterior, is the answer. However, even for advocates of nuclear flipping, a 4+ nucleus is the most dangerous time to perform this maneuver. The nucleus is very large, and the

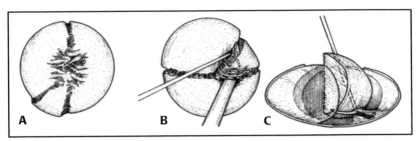

Figure 26-1. (A) Strands of the leathery posterior nucleus are maximal at the apex. (B) The surgeon passes a chopping-type instrument behind the nuclear fragment parallel to the posterior capsule. (C) The chopping instrument snaps the bridging fibers that interfere with delivering and emulsifying the nuclear fragment. (Reprinted from *Cataract Surgery*, 2nd ed, Steinert RF, The dense cataract, © 2002, with permission from Elsevier.)

capsule frequently is more fragile than usual because it is under tension. A very large capsulorrhexis would be needed to flip the nucleus, and even if this were acceptable to you with regard to later intraocular lens (IOL) implantation, phaco of a large hard nucleus in the anterior chamber will result in excessive endothelial damage.

In addressing these 4+ dense nuclei, begin with using trypan blue (Vision*Blue*, Dutch Ophthalmic Research Corporation [DORC], Rotterdam, Holland). This not only aids in performing an optimal capsulorrhexis, but also aids in keeping the edge of the anterior capsule visible during the case to avoid inadvertent damage to the rhexis and resultant capsular tear. Also, use a retentive viscoelastic liberally in the course of the surgery. You will be using a lot of phaco power and have prolonged phaco time, so protecting the endothelium is critical.

I suggest these specific steps, which have worked for me, to deal with the leathery posterior nucleus[1]:

* Bowl out the center of the nucleus. This spares the endothelium, and the large firm peripheral nucleus still provides plenty of material for the phaco tip to grab onto and hold.

* Use a chopping or finger-type instrument to break the leathery fibers. While I prefer the hook shape of my claw-shaped chopper (Rhein Medical, Tampa, Fla), there are many suitable choppers or nuclear-manipulating instruments. The maneuver is to rotate the instrument so that it is parallel to the posterior capsule. While the nuclear fragment is held by vacuum of the phaco tip and drawn partially toward the center, you pass the instrument posteriorly under the fragment, from the periphery toward the center, snapping the posterior strands (Figures 26-1B and 26-1C).

* As soon as you have any area with a visible red reflex, use this space to inject a dispersive viscoelastic behind the nucleus. This serves 3 purposes. First, it creates an artificial epinucleus to protect the posterior capsule. Second, it elevates the nucleus a little, making it easier to pass the instrument posterior to the nuclear fragments in order to snap the fiber strands. Third, it will stabilize the nuclear fragments, making it easier to position them optimally, avoiding tumbling. Do not forget to add some more viscoelastic anteriorly to protect the endothelium!

Reference

1. Steinert RF. The dense cataract. In: Steinert RF, ed. *Cataract Surgery.* 2nd ed. Philadelphia: WB Saunders; 2002.

DURING PHACO, THE POSTERIOR CAPSULE IS TRAMPOLINING MORE THAN USUAL. HOW SHOULD I PROCEED?

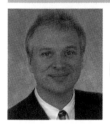

Barry S. Seibel, MD

Phacoemulsification is ideally performed in a stable and deep anterior chamber with nothing but mobilized nuclear fragments entering the phaco tip. Anterior chamber instability is often a precursor to intraoperative complications and postoperative morbidity. Such instability is often heralded by fluctuations in pupil diameter, corneal dimpling, and trampolining of the posterior capsule. Upon observing any of these warning signs, you must look for causes and take corrective action.

One of the first distinctions to make is whether the chamber and capsule fluctuation is present constantly or whether it is only manifest when the occluded phaco tip is suddenly cleared (eg, when a gripped fragment is aspirated into the tip). If frequent or constant trampolining is noted, then the machine parameters are not properly set up. One must ensure an adequate baseline infusion pressure from the elevated irrigating bottle in order to provide sufficient inflow of balanced salt solution (BSS) to keep up with outflow from the anterior chamber. This balance must be set up at the beginning of the case to allow not only steady state stability, but also an adequate buffer against postocclusion surge (to be discussed later).

The bottle height must be adequate to balance outflow as described above, but you must realize that this requirement changes every time you change to a new machine memory or mode that also changes the aspiration flow rate (ie, outflow rate). Therefore, remember to increase the bottle height setting each time that the aspiration flow rate is increased, whether the increased flow rate is set in a memory or mode on the machine or whether the flow rate is increased dynamically at the machine panel during a case (ie, in order to enhance followability). Also, be aware of incisional leakage as an occult source

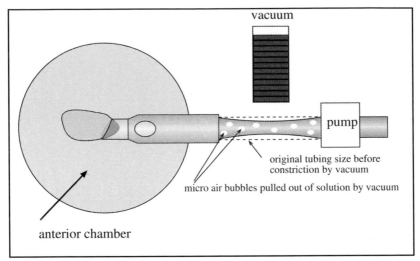

vacuum

pump

original tubing size before
constriction by vacuum

micro air bubbles pulled out of solution by vacuum

anterior chamber

Figure 27-1. Vacuum development as precursor to surge. (Reprinted with permission from Seibel BS. *Phacodynamics: Mastering the Tools and Techniques of Phacoemulsification Surgery, Fourth Edition.* Thorofare, NJ: SLACK Incorporated; 2005.)

of outflow that must be compensated for either by greater bottle height or by partially suturing an excessively large incision.

If steady state chamber stability is adequate but trampolining of the capsule is noted when the occluded phaco tip is suddenly cleared, then you are experiencing postocclusion surge. This means that potential energy within the aspiration line suddenly is added to the steady state outflow, which had previously been sufficiently limited to maintain a steady chamber. The net increase in outflow exceeds the infusion pressure capability afforded by the particular height of the irrigating bottle and the chamber becomes more shallow. This will be manifested by anterior displacement of the posterior capsule (trampolining), posterior displacement of the cornea (dimpling), and centripetal displacement of the pupil margin (constriction) (Figures 27-1 and 27-2).

The potential aspiration line energy that leads to postocclusion surge is produced by buildup of vacuum between the phaco machine pump and the occluded aspiration port of the phaco tip. The amount of energy buildup depends on the compliance of the machine's tubing, which is the change in volume divided by the change in pressure. Newer phaco machines have stiffer, less compliant tubing that resists significant volume changes with vacuum buildup. If you are using a newer machine and are still noting postocclusion surge, then the first parameter to adjust is bottle height. This should be raised to create increased infusion pressure and inflow to buffer the momentarily increased outflow due to postocclusion surge.

If chamber fluctuations and posterior capsule trampolining are still noted after raising the bottle as high as possible, the maximum commanded vacuum may be too much for your particular machine and technique. The vacuum level may need to be correspondingly decreased. Alternatively, fluidic resistors may be employed to decrease the rate of fluid egress from the anterior chamber. Such resistors include smaller bore phaco needles (including multi-bore models such as the MicroFlow [Bausch & Lomb,

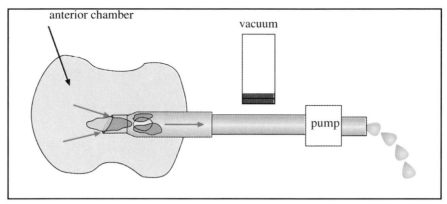

Figure 27-2. Postocclusion surge. (Reprinted with permission from Seibel BS. *Phacodynamics: Mastering the Tools and Techniques of Phacoemulsification Surgery, Fourth Edition.* Thorofare, NJ: SLACK Incorporated; 2005.)

Rochester, NY], Flare Tip [Alcon, Inc, Fort Worth, Tex], and the Cobra Tip [Surgical Designs Corp, Long Island City, NY]) (Figure 27-3). Other resistors include external devices between the phaco handpiece and the aspiration line, such as the Vacuum Surge Suppressor (STAAR Surgical, Monrovia, Calif) and the Cruise Control (STAAR Surgical). Such external devices are particularly useful for the minority of surgeons employing a bimanual microincision technique in which many infusion handpieces deliver insufficient fluid volume to single-handedly combat postocclusion surge.

In addition to inadequate baseline settings or excessive incisional outflow, other causes of anterior chamber instability may be traced to various pathologies. Weak zonules can lead to capsule trampolining in the absence of corneal dimpling or pupil constriction; watch out for this phenomenon in cases of pseudoexfoliation or prior eye trauma. Moderate to highly myopic eyes can also exhibit such signs of weak or compliant zonules. Similar effects can be noted in eyes status postvitrectomy due to the absence of the more viscous vitreous and the surface tension of an intact hyaloid face. The aforementioned measures can ameliorate consequent capsular trampolining even though they may not eliminate it entirely.

Several surgical techniques can further combat posterior capsule trampolining. Hydrodelineation creates an artifactual epinucleus that can stabilize the capsular bag during disassembly and emulsification of the endonucleus. A similar effect can be achieved with ophthalmic viscosurgical devices by creating a pseudoepinucleus using a Soft Shell technique as described by Steve A. Arshinoff, MD: a cohesive ophthalmic viscosurgical device (OVD) core is quickly evacuated, but the dispersive OVD shell can maintain capsular structure for most of the case.

Conclusion

Trampolining of the capsular bag signals a higher potential for complications. The surgeon must be vigilant for signs of this problem and employ countermeasures as described above to restabilize the anterior chamber and increase the odds of a successful outcome.

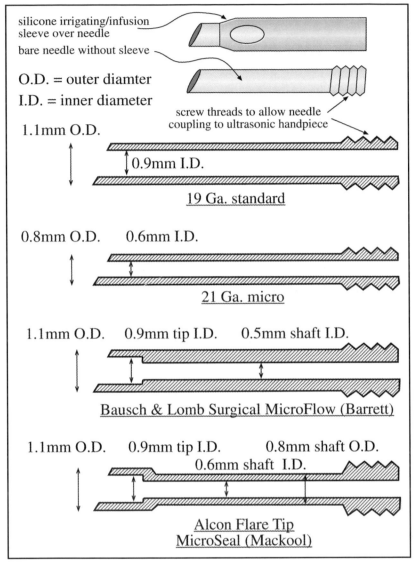

Figure 27-3. Phaco needle designs. (Reprinted with permission from Seibel BS. *Phacodynamics: Mastering the Tools and Techniques of Phacoemulsification Surgery, Fourth Edition.* Thorofare, NJ: SLACK Incorporated; 2005.)

Bibliography

Arshinoff SA. Dispersive-cohesive viscoelastic soft shell technique. *J Cataract Refract Surg.* 1999;25(2):167-173.
Seibel BS. *Phacodynamics: Mastering the Tools and Techniques of Phacoemulsification Surgery, Fourth Edition.* Thorofare, NJ: SLACK Incorporated; 2005.

WHAT ARE THE
EARLIEST INTRAOPERATIVE CLUES OF
POSTERIOR CAPSULAR RUPTURE?

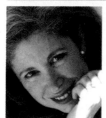

Lisa B. Arbisser, MD

Vitreous loss is inevitable in cataract surgery. Ironically, vitreous loss is inversely proportional to the surgeon's volume. Although rare, our index of suspicion must be high to appreciate the early signs of complications and to allow optimum correction. Damage control and avoidance of collateral damage are the keys to excellent outcomes. Vitreous traction intraoperatively as well as postoperatively must be scrupulously avoided because subsequent retinal detachment is definitely associated with poor visual results.

Preoperative history and slit-lamp examination may identify trauma-associated cataractogenesis. Posterior capsule or zonular apparatus integrity may be compromised as evidenced by rapid development of a hypermature cataract or lens subluxation. Vitreous prolapsing through the zonules is an obvious clue. Intraoperatively, a subtle bounce of the iris diaphragm, change in anterior chamber depth, or change in pupil size may result from sudden redistribution of fluid associated with a break in the posterior capsule at any time. Once the nucleus is mobilized after hydrodissection, the loss of rotational ability should be interpreted as evidence that capsule integrity has been breached. During phacoemulsification, assuming phaco parameters are accurate and there is no warning bell signaling tip occlusion, the loss of followability of lens material may be due to vitreous insinuated between lens fragments and the phaco tip. The collagen fibrils of vitreous cannot be "phacoed" and should not be aspirated because retinal traction will occur. In addition, tilting of the lens equator signals impending loss of lens material into the posterior segment. An unusually clear view to the posterior segment in a limited area is an open capsule. These signs demand attention. Anything between the lips of a sutureless incision will prevent an internal seal from forming. In a well-constructed wound that fails

Table 28-1

Handy Anterior Vitrectomy Kit

- Vitrector set
- MVR blade
- Chamber maintainer
- Washed Kenalog (instructions)
- Lidocaine for subconjunctival injection
- Sub-Tenon's cannula
- Cautery
- 8-0 Vicryl suture (unless sutureless technique is used with 23 gauge)
- Kansas forceps, vectis, or spoon
- Caliper
- Miochol E
- Conjunctival scissor
- Alternate implants
- Ocular hypotensives
- Antibiotic prophylaxis of choice

to prove watertight, after irrigating the tunnel to eliminate debris, search for an occult strand of incarcerated vitreous. A peaked pupil or movements of the pupil edge with remote touch are classic warning signs.

If rupture of either capsule or zonules is identified, go to foot position zero in order to stop phaco or irrigation and aspiration (I&A). Maintain chamber stability by not withdrawing the instrument until dispersive viscoelastic can be placed through the side-port to prevent chamber collapse. Inspect and introspect to call up the right decision tree and mobilize the staff and necessary equipment.

Topical anesthesia is not incompatible with managing complications. Without pain receptors, the vitreous cannot "hurt." Topical and/or intracameral anesthesia may not require supplementation except when the pars plana incision is employed or the wound needs to be significantly enlarged. A bleb of subconjunctival lidocaine 2% over the intended scleral incision prior to incising a fornix flap for pars plana incision is appropriate. Avoid reintroduction of intracameral unpreserved 1% xylocaine. Although there is evidence of no permanent damage to the neuroretina, transient amaurosis will result. This can be frightening to both the patient and the surgeon. Intravenous sedation helps the patient cooperate or pass the time more quickly. A calm voice (vocal local) and an operating room team prepared for vitrectomy (Table 28-1) help minimize patient anxiety. If these measures fail and the patient loses the ability to cooperate, akinesia may be required. First, be sure incisions are closed, avoiding loss of the anterior chamber. Use of a Masket cannula (Rhein) to perform sub-Tenon's or parabulbar block reduces the risk of retrobulbar hemorrhage.

If there is a posterior capsule break, no matter how round, there is risk for extension unless converted to a true posterior continuous curvilinear capsulorrhexis (PCCC). If it is too large, too peripheral, or if the vitreous has already prolapsed, the area is compartmentalized with viscoelastic.

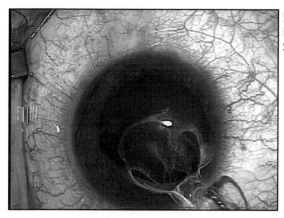

Figure 28-1. Particulate identification with intracameral-washed Kenalog. (Courtesy of Scott Burk, MD.)

If lens fragments have fallen below the posterior capsule, I discipline myself to leave them for later vitreoretinal fellowship-trained management. Although viscolevitation may prove successful, the risk of causing harm to the retina or leaving significant lens material hiding laterally exceeds the benefit of avoiding a secondary intervention if subspecialty care is readily available. If pursued, a viscoelastic cannula is placed through a pars plana incision under the sunken lens fragment and a cushion of viscoelastic is used to prevent further descent. The cannula tip is then used to levitate the fragment up into the anterior chamber.[1] It is never clear, however, in my mind where the vitreous starts and ends in this process. Under no circumstances should a phaco tip, vectis, or any other instrument be used to fish for fragments in the posterior segment, and never irrigate the posterior segment because a retinal tear will likely occur.[2]

If lens fragments are above the posterior capsule but still under the iris, they must be raised into the anterior chamber with viscoelastic from an anterior approach or dialed, lifted, or cantilevered up with a cystotome or other instrument. This is facilitated by pupil stretch, microsphincterotomies, or capsulorrhexis (CCC) enlargement. Relaxation incisions are a last resort because the integrity of the CCC is important for later implant placement.

Now identify the whereabouts of vitreous with intracameral Kenalog (Bristol-Myers-Squibb, New York, NY) particles (Figure 28-1). I prefer to wash out the diluents to remove preservatives as described by Burk (see Question 32).[3] Do not sweep incisions or use cellulose sponges to identify vitreous. These maneuvers cause significant remote retinal traction.

I would continue phaco only if there is no admixture of vitreous and lens material. The rent in the posterior capsule can be covered with a lens glide or with the iris itself by instilling Miochol E (Novartis) intracamerally to keep fragments from falling through. Fragments are removed within a viscoelastic sandwich with low flow parameters, a low bottle height, and a noncontinuous ultrasound strategy such as Burst Mode. Make sure that flow is established before engaging ultrasound to prevent wound burn in this viscoelastic-filled environment. Nonpreserved intracameral epinephrine is used to redilate the pupil as needed.

Convert to extracapsular cataract extraction (ECCE) if there is admixture of vitreous with lens material or possibly if there is a large dense fragment remaining. The vitrector can be used from the anterior approach in a "dry" fashion without irrigation to extricate lens material from vitreous. Never allow the eye to collapse. Maintain it with viscoelastic. If lens material can be broken into small chunks removable through a <4-mm incision, employ the original incision. If not, the clear corneal incision should be irrigated, closed, and abandoned as a super paracentesis. Construct an appropriate scleral or limbal incision superiorly. Do not employ standard extracapsular external pressure, which may result in expression of vitreous or retina. The nucleus is floated out with viscoelastic or guided out with a nonirrigating vectis or spoon within a viscoelastic sandwich protecting the corneal endothelium. Incisions are closed watertight.

Once nuclear lens fragments are removed, remove any prolapsed vitreous. Because vitreous always follows a gradient of high to low pressure, the pars plana approach proves most efficient and safe. Technique details are discussed elsewhere, but I employ irrigation through the anterior side-port and the vitrector on highest cut rate and low suction through an incision made with an MVR blade 3.5 mm posterior to the limbus. Repeated Kenalog identification confirms the endpoint of removal to below the plane of the posterior capsule. Suture the incision with 8-0 Vicryl if 20-gauge instruments are used.

I then either use a "dry" manual technique to remove residual cortex or I use the vitrector with a setting of "irrigation-aspiration-cut" (I&A-cut). This setting, available on all anterior segment machines, unlike the default irrigation-cut-aspiration intended for vitreous removal, allows followability of cortex in foot position two. I will not chew up remaining capsule with this setting and it allows me to cut vitreous in foot position three if necessary. This is safer for cortex removal than using the standard I&A handpiece.

Once the anterior segment is clear of lens and vitreous, decide on the location and style of lens implant (intraocular lens [IOL]). Bag placement should be confined to cases with a true PCCC and zonular integrity (with or without a capsular tension ring). I prefer a single-piece acrylic lens. Lacking a secure posterior capsule, my next best placement is to sulcus implant and optic capture a 3-piece foldable lens through the intact CCC. Lacking this anatomy, I must decide if the lens can be secure when free in the sulcus. Due to a large sulcus or lack of adequate capsule support, I have seen too many IOLs referred with subluxation or decentration. I might iris fixate in the sulcus, but if it has been a long case or there is already a larger incision, I do not hesitate to opt for a 4-point fixation Kelman-style anterior chamber lens. I create a vitrector superior iridectomy. I do not practice scleral fixation in this setting.

Miochol E is instilled for miosis and OVD carefully removed with the vitrector on I&A-cut mode, watching for vitreous presentation. Incision integrity is confirmed. In addition to routine topical medications, I use one-time oral fourth-generation fluoroquinolone prophylaxis and oral acetazolamide pressure prophylaxis immediately postop. Candid discussions with patients and close follow-up, including mandatory indented retinal exam in the postoperative period and prompt referral for definitive care of significant retained lens fragments, are mandatory.

Preparation results in effective crisis management. With maintenance of good intraocular pressure, protection of vulnerable tissues, and avoidance of vitreous traction throughout the case, we can provide our patients with a clean anterior segment, a secure implant, and an excellent visual outcome.[4]

References

1. Chang DF, Packard RB. Posterior assisted levitation for nucleus retrieval using Viscoat after posterior capsule rupture. *J Cataract Refract Surg.* 2003;29(10):1860-1865.
2. Moore JK, Scott IU, Flynn HW, et al. Retinal detachment in eyes undergoing pars plana vitrectomy for removal of retained lens fragments. *Ophthalmology.* 2003;110:709-714.
3. Burk SE, Da Mata AP, Snyder ME, et al. Visualizing vitreous using Kenalog suspension. *J Cataract Refract Surg.* 2003;29:645-651.
4. Arbisser LB, Charles S, Howcroft M, Werner L. Management of vitreous loss and dropped nucleus during cataract surgery. *Ophthalmol Clin N Am.* 2006;19(4):495-506.

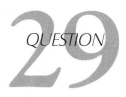

THE CAPSULAR BAG IS UNEXPECTEDLY MOBILE DURING PHACO. WHEN SHOULD I IMPLANT A CAPSULAR TENSION RING AND WHICH SIZE SHOULD I USE?

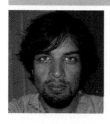

Iqbal Ike K. Ahmed, MD, FRCSC

The best management approach to weak zonules during phaco is aimed toward maintaining a small-incision closed system, avoiding vitreous prolapse, preventing further iatrogenic zonular damage, and maintaining the integrity of the capsular bag for in-the-bag posterior chamber intraocular lens (PCIOL) implantation.

The first decision is to determine whether the case can continue with a modified phaco technique and adjunctive devices or whether the capsulo-zonular apparatus is so severely compromised that one needs to convert to an extracapsular cataract extraction (ECCE) with or without a pars plana posterior-assisted levitation (PAL) technique. I reserve this only for the most profound cases of zonular instability or if there is a capsular tear present.

In most cases, phaco can be safely continued with the use of any one or combination of the following devices: iris/capsular retractors (Figure 29-1), the capsular tension segment (CTS) (not approved by the US Food and Drug Administration) (Figure 29-2), the capsular tension ring (CTR) (Figure 29-3), or the modified CTR (M-CTR) (Figure 29-4). It is important to understand that the roles of these devices are 2-fold: they provide intraoperative support for phaco and they provide long-term postoperative support for an endocapsular PCIOL.

Figure 29-1. Iris retractors placed at the capsulorrhexis edge to support localized area of zonular weakness

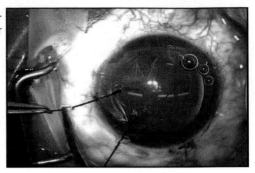

Figure 29-2. The capsular tension segment (CTS).

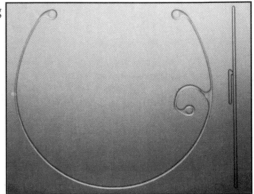

Figure 29-3. The capsular tension ring (CTR).

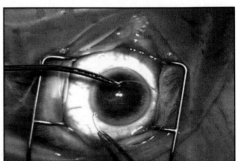

Figure 29-4. The modified capsular tension ring (M-CTR).

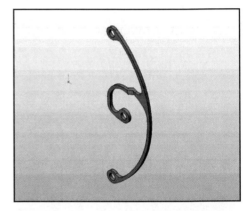

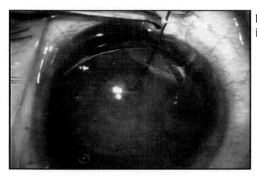

Figure 29-5. CTS in positioned support by inverted iris retractor.

Iris retractors, which have been designed to open a small pupil, or capsular retractors, which are modified for capsular placement, can be of immense use during these weak zonular cases. Every operating room should have these devices available for emergency situations. I find that iris retractors work fine for this purpose, although many surgeons have also used the specially designed capsular retractors. The iris/capsular retractors are placed on the capsulorrhexis edge to support the anterior capsule and center the capsular bag. As many retractors as required are used to support the area(s) of zonular weakness. They act as "synthetic zonules" that can be placed at any time during the procedure and are particularly useful during completion of the continuous curvilinear capsulorrhexis (CCC). The downsides of these devices include the potential for creating an anterior capsule tear at the point of contact and the possibility of the hooks becoming dislodged during the procedure. In addition, these retractors do not expand the capsular equator. This can lead to great difficulty during phaco and during cortical stripping and may fail to prevent aspiration of a lax capsule.

The CTR does an excellent job of expanding the capsular equator; however, it can be tricky to insert (see below). In cases of mild zonular weakness, the CTR alone is sufficient to stabilize the capsular bag; however, CTRs will not recenter or support the bag in cases of moderate or severe zonular instability. In these more advanced cases, sutured devices should be used.

The CTS can provide the dual benefits of a CTR and capsule retractors and can be easily placed with the capsular bag at any time during the case (Figure 29-5). To fixate the CTS to the sclera during surgery, an iris retractor is placed through the fixation eyelet.

For me, the selection and the timing of device placement depends primarily on 2 factors. The first is the degree of focal zonulopathy, which is quantified according to the number of clock hours of zonular dialysis and/or a qualitative assessment of generalized zonular weakness (eg, any phacodonesis?). The second factor is the density of the cataract. I simply grade the zonulopathy as being either minimal, mild, moderate, or severe (Table 29-1).

I use a CTR in all cases with any zonular instability, unless there is an anterior or posterior capsular tear or discontinuity. I use a larger size ring (ie, 13 mm) in most cases because this provides greater centrifugal force and ensures adequate overlap of the end terminals.

The main question with CTRs is one of timing, and this will depend on the lens density. The CTR can be placed anytime after completion of the capsulorrhexis and should be inserted as early as is necessary. CTR placement prior to phaco can be accomplished

	Table 29-1	
	Zonulopathy Severity Grading	
Minimal	No overt dialysis	Minimal phacodonesis
Mild	<4 clock hours of dialysis	Mild phacodonesis
Moderate	4 to 8 clock hours of dialysis	Moderate phacodonesis
Severe	>8 clock hours of dialysis	Severe phacodonesis

safely in softer and medium density cataracts. One key suggestion in placing a CTR before phaco is to perform viscodissection rather than hydrodissection of the nucleus. Using a cohesive ophthalmic viscosurgical device (OVD) will cleave the cortical-capsular attachments, create space for CTR implantation, and provide enough lubrication to facilitate dialing the CTR into position.

In contrast, with a very dense lens, one needs to weigh the risks and benefits of early versus late insertion because of the potential for the CTR to tear the zonules or the capsule as it is implanted. This is because of the paucity of cortex and epinucleus with dense, bulky cataracts. In these cases, I try to delay implantation until the nucleus has been grooved and debulked so as to create more room within the bag for dialing the CTR into position. In order to delay CTR implantation for as long as possible, iris/capsular retractors or the CTS may be used to stabilize the capsular bag during phaco (discussed later).

CTR implantation may be performed either manually or with an injector (my preference). As it is implanted, the CTR should be directed toward the area of greatest zonular dehiscence in order to stress the compromised areas as little as possible. A Kuglen or similar hook can provide counter-traction if needed. In cases of advanced zonular weakness, the presence of iris/capsular retractors or the CTS can stabilize the capsular bag against the torque generated as the CTR is inserted.

Phaco Pearls

For eyes with weak zonules, I do not alter my incision in order to preserve the advantages of a temporal clear cornea approach. If the zonular dialysis is temporal, I place the appropriate device needed to support this area beneath the incision.

In terms of OVD, I prefer a soft-shell technique. A dispersive OVD is used to coat the corneal endothelium and to cover the area of zonular dialysis, while a central cohesive core stabilizes the anterior chamber (AC). In the most severe cases, extra syringes of OVD will probably be necessary. As nuclear emulsification is nearing completion, placing Healon 5 (Advanced Medical Optics, Santa Ana, Calif) within the capsular bag can prevent the tendency for the capsular bag to collapse inward.

The advantages of a capsulorrhexis are well known, but this is even more critical in these cases. The capsulorrhexis ideally should be centered, round, and 5 mm in diameter. This size is large enough to facilitate lens removal and to prevent postoperative capsular phimosis and is also adequately sized for placement of iris/capsular retractors or a CTS. This diameter opening also permits continuous edge overlap of the intraocular lens (IOL) optic.

In cases of moderate to severe zonulopathy, it is important to stabilize the capsular bag with the appropriate device prior to phaco; otherwise, there is increased risk of vitreous prolapse, loss of nuclear fragments, or posterior capsular rupture.

In terms of phaco technique, if the lens is soft with a healthy cornea and a deep AC, I prefer to flip the nucleus and perform supracapsular phaco. If the circumstances are not appropriate for a phaco flip technique, an endocapsular vertical phaco chop is preferred. It is helpful to lower the fluidics and slow down the procedure in these cases.

It is essential that there be no loss of AC during the procedure, particularly during instrument exchange (ie, after phaco or after cortical aspiration). If this should occur, there is a significant risk of vitreous prolapse through/around the weak zonule. Balanced salt solution (BSS) or an OVD should be injected to prevent loss of AC at these times.

If vitreous prolapse is present preoperatively or occurs intraoperatively, a vitrectomy (either bimanual through limbal paracentesis incisions or pars plana with AC infusion as indicated) should be performed prior to continuation of phaco. However, the vitrectomy should not be initiated until after the capsular bag has been adequately supported and stabilized with the appropriate device. This avoids the potential for posterior dislocation of the nucleus during the vitrectomy.

Device Selection Guidelines

MINIMAL ZONULOPATHY

In these cases, a simple CTR is sufficient and this may be implanted either early on or at the end of the procedure. Because the zonules are only minimally affected, simply employing a phaco technique that minimizes zonular stress should alone suffice. The indication for the CTR is to provide postoperative IOL centration and support.

MILD ZONULOPATHY

Again, a simple CTR is sufficient. In these cases, it is advantageous to place the CTR as early as possible. I sometimes like to have an iris/capsular retractor placed over the area of dialysis to stabilize this area and to provide counter-traction during CTR insertion. The retractors can either be left in until after IOL implantation or removed after CTR implantation. A sutured capsular tension device, such as the CTS or M-CTR, is usually not needed in these cases.

MODERATE ZONULOPATHY

These cases do require a sutured device—either the CTS or M-CTR. I employ iris/capsular retractors while performing the CCC to re-center the capsular bag and to provide counter-traction. I then place a CTS over the area of zonular dialysis and place an iris retractor within the CTS to support the capsular bag in this quadrant. A CTR is then implanted after which phaco can be performed safely in a well-supported environment.

The CTS can be permanently sutured to the sclera using 9-0 polypropylene. Alternatively, the M-CTR may be used; however, it is difficult to implant this device early in the case prior to phaco, and thus one must rely only on iris/capsular retractors until the lens has been evacuated.

SEVERE ZONULOPATHY

The same principles apply as with moderate zonulopathy cases, but typically 2 CTS devices are required 180 degrees apart. Alternatively, the double-eyelet M-CTR may be used.

Intraocular Lens Selection and Placement

In-the-bag PCIOL placement is by far the ideal location. If the capsular bag has been well supported with a CTR with or without a sutured device (ie, CTS or M-CTR), this should be a stable environment in the long term. I prefer an acrylic PCIOL, which has less tendency for anterior capsular opacification and capsular contracture, which can lead to postoperative decentration.

Although it may be tempting to place a PCIOL in the sulcus in these cases, I generally avoid this. Unless the zonular deficiency is supported, sulcus IOLs are also at risk for postoperative decentration. Other alternatives, should an in-the-bag PCIOL be deemed risky, include an iris-sutured PCIOL, an iris-claw artisan aphakic IOL, or an AC IOL.

Postoperative Monitoring

Postoperatively, one must carefully monitor the eye for capsular contracture. If this occurs, Nd:YAG laser anterior capsule relaxing incisions should be performed in order to release the tension and spread the contracting forces so as to avoid IOL decentration.

If postoperative IOL decentration does occur, the lens should be surgically repositioned as soon as possible. The presence of a CTR provides one with the option to pass a polypropylene suture loop under and over the CTR (needle passed through the bag to get under the CTR) so that the CTR becomes fixated to the sclera. Typically 1, 2, or even 3 fixation points may be required.

Bibliography

Ahmed IIK, Cionni RJ, Kranemann C, Crandall AS. Optimal timing of capsular tension ring implantation: a Miyake-Apple video analysis. *J Cataract Refract Surg.* 2005;31(9):1809-1813.

Bayraktar S, Alton T, Kucuksumer Y, Yilmaz OF. Capsular tension ring implantation after capsulorrhexis in phaco-emulsification of cataracts associated with pseudoexfoliation syndrome: intraoperative complications and early postoperative findings. *J Cataract Refract Surg.* 2001;27:1620-1628.

Cionni RJ, Osher RH. Management of profound zonular dialysis or weakness with a new endocapsular ring designed for scleral fixation. *J Cataract Refract Surg.* 1998;24:1299-1306.

Hasanee K, Ahmed IK. Capsular tension rings: update on endocapsular support devices. *Ophthalmol Clin North Am.* 2006;19:507-519.

Hasanee K, Butler M, Ahmed II. Capsular tension rings and related devices: current concepts. *Curr Opin Ophthalmol.* 2006;17:31-41.

WHAT SHOULD I DO WHEN
THE DIAMETER OF MY COMPLETED
CAPSULORRHEXIS IS VERY SMALL?

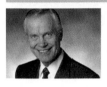

Howard V. Gimbel, MD, MPH, FRCSC, FACS

There is not much debate regarding the ideal size of a continuous curvilinear capsulor-rhexis (CCC) for standard cataract surgery with posterior chamber intraocular lens (IOL) implantation. Nishi et al have shown that there is less fibrosis and opacification of the posterior capsule if the edge of the anterior capsule opening is not allowed to touch the posterior capsule and is kept on top of the IOL.[1]

Another strong reason to keep the CCC 0.5 mm to 1 mm smaller than the optic is the ability to use rhexis fixation or optic capture by the CCC if a posterior capsule tear neces-sitates placement of the IOL in the sulcus. Lenses designed for the bag may not be stable in the sulcus and may result in uveitis-glaucoma-hyphema (UGH) syndrome, transillumina-tion defects, secondary glaucoma, or displacement of the IOL eccentrically by herniating vitreous after a YAG capsulotomy.[2] The IOL may also be displaced anteriorly against the iris and even the optic out of the pupil by an expanding Soemmering's Ring.

The characteristics of the various ophthalmic viscosurgical devices (OVD) influence the technique of capsulorrhexis. There is risk of radializing tears when using low viscosi-ty viscoelastics. However, when using the highly viscous viscoelastics, there is a tendency to make the CCC smaller than intended. Also, highly viscous viscoelastics can displace the crystalline lens and/or the iris when injected into the anterior chamber somewhat peripherally. This can result in an eccentric CCC when it is made concentric to the pupil. Inadvertently or purposefully small as well as eccentric CCCs may usually be modified to achieve centration and a more ideal size. I will review 2-stage CCC techniques that can often be used to make these modifications.[3]

Figure 30-1. Two-staged CCC is started with a tangential cut on one side of the opening with a Vannas scissors.

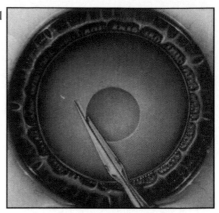

Figure 30-2. Forceps are used to enlarge the original capsulotomy by removing a strip or ribbon of additional capsule.

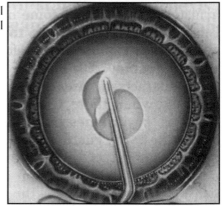

Two-staged techniques may be performed before phacoemulsification, after nucleus or cortical removal, or after IOL placement. Small CCCs can make it difficult to remove subincisional cortex using coaxial irrigation and aspiration (I/A). Enlarging a small CCC can make removal possible without changing to bimanual I/A or other techniques such as bent cannulas or angled I/A tips.

Small capsular openings are enlarged in a second step in the following manner. Additional highly viscous viscoelastic is used to flatten the anterior capsule and to lift it off the IOL or the lens if it is still there. Capsule scissors are then used to make a tangential snip on one side of the opening (Figure 30-1). Care should be taken to prevent the side of the capsule opening from folding as the scissors make a cut in the edge because this results in a V cut with a propensity to tear radially. Complete closure of the scissors should also be avoided because the point of the scissors may cause an irregularity at the end of the cut, making it difficult to properly start the next tear. Capsule forceps are then used to grasp the start of the new flap to create a larger curvilinear tear by removing a strip or ribbon of additional capsule (Figure 30-2). Multiple regraspings of the secondary tear with attention to the vector forces will result in a controlled continuous tear of desired width and length (Figure 30-3). If the CCC is to be enlarged symmetrically, the ribbon of tissue is guided all the way around the existing CCC (Figure 30-4). Eccentric CCCs may be centered by taking additional tissue from only one side.

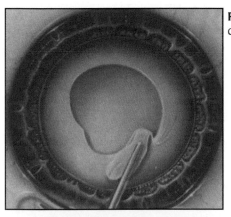

Figure 30-3. The continuous tear is extended in the desired direction.

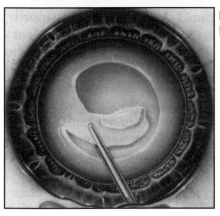

Figure 30-4. Two-staged CCC near completion, resulting in an opening of desired diameter.

A similar tearing technique can be used to blunt or turn back short inadvertent radial tears of the anterior capsular rim. Radialized tears that occur during capsulorrhexis that are too long to turn back may be managed by starting a new tear away from the radial tear to complete the capsulorrhexis from the opposite direction.

Another option for performing a 2-staged CCC as well as for the primary CCC is the use of a plasma blade.[4] It can easily start and complete the second stage and fashion an opening of ideal size and shape. It is particularly useful if fibrous bands involving the anterior capsule prevent the curvilinear tear from progressing, as this blade easily cuts through dense tissue.

Obtaining an ideal capsule opening is one of the most critical steps in cataract surgery. These second stage techniques can often rescue or improve less-than-ideal beginnings of the cataract operation.

References

1. Nishi O, Nishi K, Osakabe Y. Effect of intraocular lenses on preventing posterior capsule opacification: design versus material. *J Cataract Refract Surg.* 2004;30:2170-2176.
2. Gimbel HV, DeBroff BM. Intraocular lens optic capture. *J Cataract Refract Surg.* 2004;30:200-206.
3. Gimbel HV. Two-stage capsulorrhexis for endocapsular phacoemulsification. *J Cataract Refract Surg.* 1990;16(2):246-249.
4. Singh D. Use of the Fugo blade in complicated cases. *J Cataract Refract Surg.* 2002;28(4):573-574.

31

WHEN SHOULD AN ANTERIOR VITRECTOMY BE PERFORMED VIA THE PARS PLANA VERSUS THE LIMBUS?

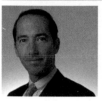

Louis D. "Skip" Nichamin, MD

I think most phaco surgeons would agree that the single most significant complication still faced today, albeit rare, is rupture of the posterior capsule and vitreous loss. Fortunately, in the setting of modern small incision surgery, if one adheres to certain fundamental principles and employs proper instrumentation and surgical technique, the vast majority of these challenging eyes will enjoy an outcome that differs little from that of an uncomplicated case.[1,2] I believe that in nearly all such cases, the utilization of a pars plana approach will greatly facilitate clean-up of the anterior segment, optimize surgeon control over the situation, and ultimately lead to far better patient outcomes.[3]

The guiding principles for this complication include quick recognition of the problem, avoidance of ocular hypotony, and maintenance of a closed-chamber environment. This requires the use of watertight incisions. As such, a much lower rate and volume of infusion may be used, thereby reducing intraocular turbulence. To further enhance control of the intraocular environment and reduce vitreoretinal traction, a separated or bimanual vitrectomy should be utilized. In this way, the location and vector force of the infusion are displaced from the point where one is attempting to delicately remove vitreous. An acceptable approach would be to place both instruments through limbal incisions (Figure 31-1).

I would submit to you, however, that greater efficiency and even safety may be achieved by placing the vitrectomy cutter through a pars plana incision (Figure 31-2). This allows the surgeon to "pull down" prolapsed vitreous from the anterior chamber, markedly reducing the amount of vitreous that is removed from the eye. When working from the limbus and bringing vitreous up, it is much more difficult to find an "end point," and

Figure 31-1. Bimanual vitrectomy performed through limbal incisions. (Reprinted with permission from Nichamin LD. Posterior capsular rupture and vitreous loss: advanced approaches. In: Chang DF, ed. *Phaco Chop: Mastering Techniques, Optimizing Technology, and Avoiding Complications.* Thorofare, NJ: SLACK Incorporated; 2004.)

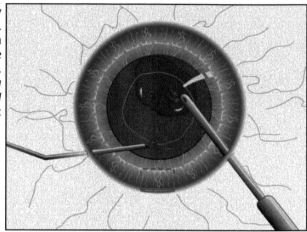

Figure 31-2. Bimanual vitrectomy with vitreous cutter placed through the pars plana incision. (Reprinted with permission from Nichamin LD. Posterior capsular rupture and vitreous loss: advanced approaches. In: Chang DF, ed. *Phaco Chop: Mastering Techniques, Optimizing Technology, and Avoiding Complications.* Thorofare, NJ: SLACK Incorporated; 2004.)

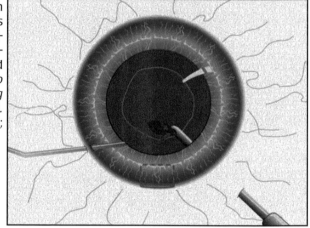

one often unintentionally removes a considerable portion of the vitreous body and must then deal with a hypotonus eye.

Another significant advantage to working through a pars plana incision is the enhanced access one has to residual lens material. Cortex, epinucleus, and even medium density nucleus may be removed with the vitrectomy instrument by increasing vacuum and reducing the cutting rate. When addressing vitreous, the highest cut rate is used with the lowest possible vacuum that allows for tissue removal. Such vacuum settings are typically in the range of 100 mm Hg to 150 mm Hg, and modern vitrectors are now capable of cutting at rates of 1500 cuts per minute. In this way, a more complete "clean-up" may be achieved, reducing secondary complications such as increased intraocular pressure (IOP), inflammation, and cystoid macular edema (CME).

It goes without saying that care and effort must be directed toward the learning and acquisition of any new surgical technique, but in reality the pars plana approach is quite straightforward. Typically, one first takes down the conjunctiva and applies light cautery at the site of the intended sclerotomy, although some surgeons will incise directly through the conjunctiva. The cardinal meridia should be avoided due to increased vascularity. Given that the posterior capsule is open, infusion may be placed through a limbal paracentesis incision or through a second pars incision. The exact clock hour of the vitrectomy incision should be selected based on the remaining capsular anatomy and how best one may approach and access remaining lens material.

The pars plana is located between 3.0 mm and 4.0 mm posterior to the limbus, so most commonly the incision is placed 3.5 mm from the limbus, though an adjustment may be made for unusual axial lengths. Depending upon surgeon preference, wounds are created to accommodate either 19-gauge or 20-gauge instruments. A dedicated disposable microvitreoretinal (MVR) knife should be used to create properly sized and therefore watertight incisions for both pars plana and limbal incisions. In creating the pars plana incision, the MVR blade is held perpendicular to the scleral surface and usually oriented in a nonradial fashion. The blade is directed toward the center of the globe with a simple in-and-out motion.

Care should be taken in both cleaning and closing the pars plana incision. Choices for suture closure vary but would include 9-0 nylon or 8-0 Vicryl. Recently, 25-gauge instrumentation has become available that, in some settings, may allow for sutureless surgery. Normal insertion, however, requires a firm globe. These instruments could be used in an open-globe/complicated setting by first creating small incisions with a sharp blade as opposed to the usual trochar system. One downside is their lack of tensile rigidity and, therefore, an ability to manipulate the position of the globe.

Is there ever a role for an anterior or limbal approach? In my opinion, this would occur if there is only a tiny breach in the capsule with a very limited amount of prolapsing vitreous, such as one occasionally finds near the end of what seemed to be an uncomplicated case. For example, the finding of a peaked pupil almost always indicates that a vitreous strand has come forward through an undetected capsular or zonular defect. If the pupil can be kept reasonably small with a miotic agent, then the prolapsing wick may either be simply swept back using an instrument placed through a side-port incision or a bimanual limbal technique may be used as depicted in Figure 31-1.

Prudence would dictate that a pars plana vitrectomy should not be performed for the first time while under duress during a live complication, but rather carefully studied and first practiced in a lab setting. I sincerely believe that the community standard regarding this technique is currently undergoing a significant change, and many vitreoretinal surgeons now endorse these thoughts. Finally, if a significant vitrectomy was required, the patient should undergo a thorough retinal exam postoperatively, and if the operating surgeon is not fully comfortable in this regard, a referral to a posterior segment surgeon ought to be made in a timely fashion.

References

1. Chang DF. Strategies for managing posterior capsular rupture. In: Chang DF, ed. *Phaco Chop: Mastering Techniques, Optimizing Technology, and Avoiding Complications.* Thorofare, NJ: SLACK Incorporated; 2004.
2. Nichamin LD. Prevention pearls and damage control. In: Fishkind WJ, ed. *Complications in Phacoemulsification.* New York, NY: Thieme; 2002:260-270.
3. Nichamin LD. Posterior capsular rupture and vitreous loss: advanced approaches. In: Chang DF, ed. *Phaco Chop: Mastering Techniques, Optimizing Technology, and Avoiding Complications.* Thorofare, NJ: SLACK Incorporated; 2004.

WHEN AND HOW DO I STAIN THE VITREOUS WITH INTRACAMERAL KENALOG?

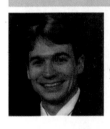

Scott E. Burk, MD, PhD

All anterior segment surgeons must occasionally face vitreous. Virtually invisible and exceptionally unwelcome, vitreous in the anterior segment makes surgery more difficult and is associated with serious intraoperative and postoperative complications. Fortunately, meticulous vitreous clean-up can reduce the incidence of many vision-threatening complications associated with vitreous loss.[1] Unfortunately, over 80% of ophthalmologists surveyed have completed surgery only to find vitreous incarceration postoperatively.[2] The main reason for this alarming statistic is that we just cannot see vitreous at the operating microscope. Until recently, surgeons were forced to use indirect clues to look for vitreous gel in the anterior chamber. Kenalog suspension (triamcinolone acetonide [TA])* solves this problem.[3]

Indications

Kenalog may be used in the anterior chamber to highlight vitreous known to be present, to check for suspected vitreous, or to confirm that an adequate vitrectomy has been performed and that all of the vitreous has been cleared from the anterior chamber (Figure 32-1). It must be noted, however, that intraocular administration of Kenalog is an "off label" use.

---

*There are various companies that produce TA. Our experience is with Kenalog-40 supplied by Bristol-Myers Squibb, New York, NY. I will refer to triamcinolone and Kenalog interchangeably; however, each surgeon should verify that their intended TA is designated as an injectable suspension and that formulation is the same as Kenalog.

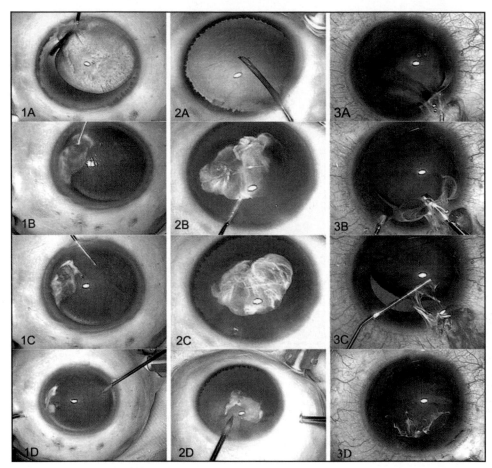

Figure 32-1. (1) Sequential images in a cadaver eye demonstrating the use of Kenalog suspension for visualizing vitreous location and removal: (A) creation of a zonular dialysis; (B) injection of Kenalog into the prolapsed vitreous gel; (C) rinsing the anterior chamber to remove a small amount of unbound Kenalog particles; (D) visualizing the removal of vitreous by a limited pars plana vitrectomy. (2) Sequential images in a cadaver eye demonstrating the use of Kenalog suspension for visualizing vitreous dynamics and assisting vitrectomy: (A) creating an intentional tear in the posterior capsule; (B) injection of Kenalog into the vitreous gel demonstrating expansion of fluid pockets; (C) Kenalog highlights the extent of vitreous prolapse; (D) visualizing the removal of vitreous by a limited pars plana vitrectomy. (3) Sequential images in an eye with a traumatic cataract, zonular dialysis, and vitreous prolapse demonstrating the use of Kenalog suspension for visualizing vitreous location and assisting vitrectomy: (A) injection of Kenalog into the anterior chamber; (B) visualization of the vitreous gel during anterior vitrectomy; (C) visualization of residual vitreous trapped at the wound after anterior vitrectomy; (D) visualizing the removal of vitreous from the anterior chamber by a limited pars plana vitrectomy.

Preparation

We continue to prepare TA as originally described and remove the preservative by a sterile capture-wash technique. Briefly, 0.2 mL of Kenalog-40 is drawn up into a tuberculin syringe and expressed into a 5-µm filter that captures the TA particles. We then rinse and resuspend the TA with balanced salt solution (BSS). The final resuspension volume is 2 mL, giving an approximate concentration of 4 mg/mL. While our TA washing technique removes the benzyl alcohol preservative, it can be tedious, particularly when the encounter with vitreous is unexpected or the operating room staff is unfamiliar with the technique.

One of the most common questions regarding intracameral TA is, "Can the preparation be simplified?" Yes, there are 3 basic options:

1. Some surgeons simply dilute 40 mg/mL TA 1:10 with BSS. This is by far the fastest and easiest option; however, the final product will contain 0.01% benzyl alcohol preservative.

2. Other surgeons prefer a sedimentation-resuspension-dilution technique. The most conceptually simple version of this technique involves leaving a Kenalog-40 vial sitting undisturbed in the operating room. When TA is needed, the supernatant is drawn off and replaced with an equal volume of BSS. The TA is typically then diluted 1:10 in BSS. Assuming supernatant removal of 90% or greater, the final product will contain 0.001% benzyl alcohol or less.

3. Finally, preservative-free TA can be purchased from compounding pharmacies but it has a limited shelf life and is more expensive.

Each surgeon and facility will need to make their own informed decisions about the preparation technique of choice; however, I think most will ultimately use a sediment-resuspend-dilute technique to minimize cost, hassle, and preservative in the preparation.

Technique

Here at the Cincinnati Eye Institute, before our complicated cases we typically prepare 2 mL of washed Kenalog at ~4 mg/mL. Higher concentrations tend to leave too much unbound TA in the anterior chamber, whereas a larger volume of the lower concentration allows the surgeon more control over the distribution of the particles.

The Kenalog is injected directly into the substance of the vitreous to obtain maximum visualization. Dusting the surface of the gel works, but only until the dusted surface has been removed by vitrectomy at which point reinjection is necessary. I like to swirl a little Kenalog gently in the anterior chamber to get an overview of the situation, and then bury the cannula tip within the gel and make a very controlled injection. You can watch the vitreous anatomy gradually appear as the particles become entrapped. It is very important to remember that vitreous follows the pressure gradient, and if vitreous is near the wound when fluid comes out, so will vitreous. Inserting the cannula through a paracentesis rather than the phaco incision tends to reduce such reflux.

The vitrectomy should be performed in cut-irrigation-aspiration mode using a high cut rate (800+), a low aspiration rate (~20), and separate irrigation. Although not always needed, a pars plana approach (3 mm behind the limbus) can be quite helpful. Indeed in eyes with a large zonular dialysis, we often make a paracentesis, instill Kenalog, and perform the vitrectomy through the pars plana before making the phaco incision.

Finally, all eyes that undergo a vitrectomy require a dilated peripheral fundus examination in the early postoperative period to look for retinal tears.

Alternatives

Visualization of the vitreous using biostaining ophthalmic dyes has been described.[4,5] While it is true that dye is held in the vitreous briefly, dye in solution is composed of relatively small molecules that rapidly diffuse away unless it becomes bound to protein. The capsular dyes are great for binding to basement membrane proteins, but there is very little protein in the vitreous. Thus, the rapid diffusion of dye and the paucity of protein to bind to in the vitreous (compared to elsewhere in the eye) result in an unacceptably low signal-to-noise ratio. After a short time, the consequence is poorly highlighted vitreous and diffuse ocular staining.

If you imagine the vitreous as a 3-dimensional microscopic spider web, it becomes more conceptually obvious why the vitreous gel will capture and hold nearly any particulate matter (think of asteroid hyalosis). Certainly, there are alternative particulate suspensions that have been evaluated for vitreous identification.[4] The most notable of these is 11-deoxycortisol, a steroid precursor without glucocorticoid effects.[6] As expected, the suspension of 11-deoxycortisol becomes trapped in vitreous just like TA.

Nonetheless, we prefer Kenalog because it is a Food and Drug Administration (FDA)-approved medication (although not approved by the FDA for this indication). It is readily available, nontoxic, and has a 27-year track record of intraocular use.[7-10] In addition, the steroid effect stabilizes the blood-aqueous barrier and minimizes postoperative inflammation in these complicated anterior segment cases.

What if I Find Vitreous Postoperatively?

Kenalog staining has revealed that vitreous prolapse through the wound or paracentesis occurs in most cases of vitreous loss. Fortunately, vitreous stained with Kenalog is much easier to visualize and remove.

When vitreous incarceration in an incision is discovered postoperatively, the first and most important task is to determine if any vitreous is exposed to the tear film. Vitreous wicking is an open invitation for infection, and unrecognized vitreous wicking undoubtedly accounts for many cases of endophthalmitis associated with vitreous loss. If externalized vitreous is not readily apparent, try staining it. This is a situation in which I favor use of the cobalt blue filter and fluorescein sodium because it brightly highlights the gel and persistent staining is not necessary. If any externalized vitreous is detected, the patient should be taken back to the operating room for additional vitrectomy using Kenalog as needed. A brief swirl of Kenalog around the anterior chamber followed by gentle rinsing with BSS should confirm the absence of any additional vitreous in the chamber.

If there is a peaked pupil indicating vitreous incarceration, but no evidence for externalized vitreous, YAG laser vitreolysis may be considered. Small strands of vitreous may be broken, but the surgeon must take care to use the minimum energy required to disrupt the strand. Thick vitreous strands will typically necessitate a return trip to the operating room for additional vitrectomy where Kenalog may be used to enhance visualization. In either case, it is important not to leave the eye with vitreous traction. To do so only invites cystoid macular edema and retinal tears.

Questions

To date, 2 questions about Kenalog-assisted vitrectomy are unresolved. The first regards the method of preparation and the effects of benzyl alcohol preservative on the intraocular structures. The use of preservative-free or washed TA makes intuitive sense, but it is not clear that the removal of the benzyl alcohol preservative is necessary. Indeed, the most recent study comparing "off the shelf" TA versus vehicle-removed/resuspended TA in a rabbit model found no difference in corneal thickness, endothelial cell count, or endothelial cell viability. The only difference identified was by scanning electron microscopy, which showed fewer microvilli on the endothelial cells that received "off the shelf" TA.[11] The significance of this is yet to be determined.

The second question relates to the probability of steroid-induced glaucoma. Increased intraocular pressure (IOP) after intravitreal injection of TA is well known to our vitreoretinal colleagues. Indeed, the amount of steroid deposited correlates both with the percentage of patients experiencing elevated IOP and with the severity of the rise in pressure.

Although it is certainly possible that an eye may develop glaucoma after undergoing TA-assisted anterior vitrectomy, we have not observed this complication. Furthermore, the risk of steroid-induced glaucoma seems to be minimal because we use only a small amount of TA and remove the majority of it along with the vitreous gel.

Conclusion

TA has proven to be an invaluable tool for visualizing vitreous in the anterior chamber and has become a routine part of our practice for complicated cataract cases, especially in eyes with large or traumatic zonular dialyses. Kenalog suspension is so useful for identifying vitreous that we believe it should be as easily available to the surgeon as viscoelastic.

Pearls

* Vitreous behaves like a microscopic 3-dimensional web enveloping pockets of fluid.
* TA highlights the exposed web strands but does not enter intact pockets unless specifically introduced.
* Highly syneretic vitreous is a collapsed web and captures less TA.

* Vitreous follows a pressure gradient. Any fluid leak will carry nearby vitreous along to the incision.

* Avoid the area of incisional vitreous prolapse and inject TA from a paracentesis to minimize reflux.

* Viscoelastic occupies space and tends to exclude both vitreous and TA.

* Shake the TA suspension immediately before using!!!

* Always examine the peripheral retina after a vitrectomy.

Acknowledgments

It is with great appreciation that I acknowledge my colleagues who made this work possible: Andrea P. Da Mata, MD, PhD; Robert H. Osher, MD; and Robert J. Cionni, MD.

References

1. Spigelman AV, Lindstrom RL, Nichols BD, Lindquist TD. Visual results following vitreous loss and primary lens implantation. *J Cataract Refract Surg.* 1989;15:201-204.
2. AAO Spotlight on Cataract 2006 Audience Response questions.
3. Burk SE, Da Mata AP, Snyder ME, Schneider S, Osher RH, Cionni RJ. Visualizing vitreous using Kenalog suspension. *J Cataract Refract Surg.* 2003;29:645-651.
4. Burk SE, Da Mata AP, Snyder ME, Rosa RH Jr, Foster RE. Indocyanine green-assisted peeling of the retinal internal limiting membrane. *Ophthalmology.* 2000;107:2010-2014.
5. Cacciatori M, Chadha V, Bennett HG, Singh J. Trypan blue to aid visualization of the vitreous during anterior segment surgery. *J Cataract Refract Surg.* 2006;32:389-391.
6. Kaji Y, Hiraoka T, Okamoto F, Sato M, Oshika T. Visualizing the vitreous body in the anterior chamber using 11-deoxycortisol after posterior capsule rupture in an animal model. *Ophthalmology.* 2004;111:1334-1339.
7. McCuen BW 2nd, Bessler M, Tano Y, Chandler D, Machemer R. The lack of toxicity of intravitreally administered triamcinolone acetonide. *Am J Ophthalmol.* 1981;91:785-788.
8. Hida T, Chandler D, Arena JE, Machemer R. Experimental and clinical observations of the intraocular toxicity of commercial corticosteroid preparations. *Am J Ophthalmol.* 1986;101:190-195.
9. Young S, Larkin G, Branley M, Lightman S. Safety and efficacy of intravitreal triamcinolone for cystoid macular edema in uveitis. *Clin Experiment Ophthalmol.* 2001;29:2-6.
10. Tano Y, Chandler D, Machemer R. Treatment of intraocular proliferation with intravitreal injection of triamcinolone acetonide. *Am J Ophthalmol.* 1980;90:810-816.
11. Oh JY, Wee WR, Lee JH, Kim MK. Short-term effect of intracameral triamcinolone acetonide on corneal endothelium using the rabbit model. *Eye.* 2006.

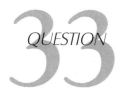
WHEN AND HOW SHOULD I IMPLANT AN INTRAOCULAR LENS IN THE CILIARY SULCUS?

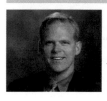

Thomas A. Oetting, MS, MD

An intraocular lens (IOL) can often be securely placed using what remains of a damaged capsule for support.[1] There are 4 typical situations: anterior capsular tear without extension, posterior capsular tear with intact anterior capsule, anterior capsular tear extending to a posterior capsular tear, and zonular dehiscence. First let us discuss how to place an IOL in the sulcus and then get to these 4 common situations.

The most important part of placing an IOL in the sulcus is getting both haptics in the sulcus.[2] The most common problem is to have one haptic in the sulcus and the other in the bag, which results in a decentered IOL (Figure 33-1).

One reason that it is hard to get both haptics in the sulcus is that the most common area of damage to the capsule is directly across from the wound. This area is vulnerable to radial tears as ophthalmic viscosurgical devices (OVD) are often running low as the capsulorrhexis passes this point, and this area is vulnerable as the phaco tip and chopper are active in this region. Unfortunately, this same area is where the leading haptic naturally flows during IOL insertion. If the capsule is damaged in this area, then the sulcus is poorly defined and the leading haptic can end up posterior to the anterior capsule rather than in the sulcus as intended.

When I am faced with capsule damage across from my wound, I will often inject the IOL into the eye and direct the leading haptic anterior to the iris in the anterior chamber to avoid the damaged capsule. I then will use Kelman McPherson forceps to place the trailing haptic into the sulcus. I then use an instrument like a Sinskey hook to rotate the IOL about 90 degrees so that the haptics are away from the damaged area. Then I take the Sinskey hook through a paracentesis, slide it over and hook onto the leading haptic, and

Figure 33-1. Decentered IOL. Superior haptic in the sulcus and inferior haptic in the bag.

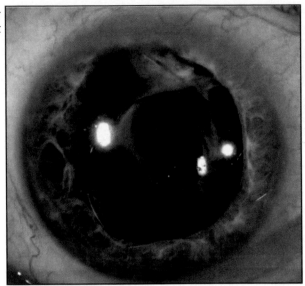

pull the haptic inside the pupil and release the haptic just under the iris into the sulcus. Defining the sulcus with a viscous dispersive viscoelastic (eg, Viscoat [Alcon, Fort Worth, Tex]) will greatly ease placement of the haptics.

The second most common problem when placing an IOL in the sulcus is using the wrong IOL design or power. The best IOL for the sulcus has a large optic that is forgiving of mild decentration and permits a better view of the peripheral retina; long haptics with an overall length that will center the IOL even in large eyes; and smooth, thin haptics to reduce chaffing of the posterior leaf of the iris. Figure 33-2[3,4] shows a single-piece acrylic lens with large square-edged haptics that was placed in the sulcus, leading to iris transillumination defects and pigmentary glaucoma. I prefer acrylic to silicone IOLs for sulcus implantation because patients with capsule trauma are at increased risk for retinal detachment and the possible use of silicone oil. I like the Alcon MA50 3-piece IOL (Fort Worth, Tex) because it has wide haptics, a large yet injectable 6.5-mm optic, and it is acrylic.

As an IOL in the sulcus is more anterior than an IOL in the bag, the power of the IOL must be reduced. In our study of 30 sulcus-based IOLs, we found that the A-constant should be lowered by about 0.8 D.[5] Other studies have had similar results, suggesting that we decrease the power of sulcus-based IOLs by 0.5 D to 1.0 D.[6]

It is very important to eliminate any vitreous in the area of IOL insertion. Vitreous streaming to the wound or to a paracentesis can cause IOL decentration. Careful bimanual anterior vitrectomy aided with Kenalog (Bristol-Myers Squibb, New York, NY) (not approved by the Food and Drug Administration for this indication) will greatly assist in the long-term stability of the IOL and retina (see Question 32).

There is no need to place a peripheral iridotomy when placing an IOL in the sulcus.

When the anterior capsule has a tear but the posterior capsule remains intact, one can often place an IOL in the bag. IOL insertion should be gentle, placing as little stress on the bag as possible. I prefer a single-piece acrylic in this case because the soft acrylic haptics, oriented 90 degrees away from the tear, create little tension on the bag, minimizing the

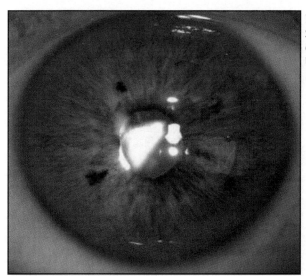

Figure 33-2. Iris transillumination defects. Single-piece acrylic in the sulcus. (Courtesy of Drs. Anthony Kuo and Robert Noecker, University of Pittsburgh.)

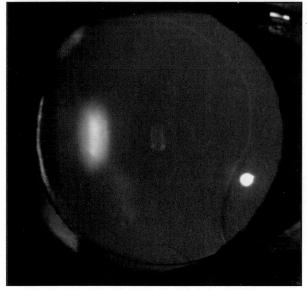

Figure 33-3. Single-piece acrylic IOL in the bag with a radial tear.

risk of extension of the tear. My experience is that the single-piece acrylic is stable in the bag with a radial tear and remains centered (Figure 33-3). The disadvantage to placing this IOL in the bag with an anterior capsular tear is that should the radial tear advance to the posterior capsule during insertion, this IOL must be removed and exchanged for a 3-piece IOL suitable for the sulcus.

When the posterior capsule is torn and the anterior capsulotomy is intact, you have 2 options for the sulcus and one for the bag. One sulcus option is to simply place the IOL in the sulcus. The second, which I often use, is to place the haptics in the sulcus as described but then use a Kuglen hook to gently prolapse the optic back into capture by a well-centered anterior capsulotomy (Figure 33-4). This optic capture is very stable and seals off the vitreous from the anterior chamber. The final option applies to stable posterior capsule tears such as round holes from a direct phaco needle strike or those tears completed with

Figure 33-4. Haptics in the sulcus and the optic is in the bag.

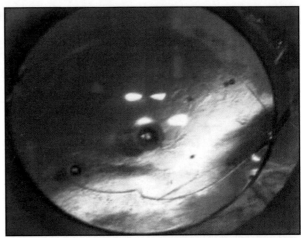

Figure 33-5. A single-piece acrylic in the bag. Round hole in the posterior capsule.

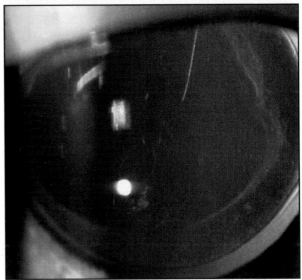

a posterior capsulorrhexis, and that is to gently place a single-piece acrylic IOL into the bag (Figure 33-5).

When the posterior and anterior capsules are both torn, it is best to seal off the area with Viscoat and to place the IOL in the sulcus as described above.

When the zonules are injured, my first thought is to try placing a capsular tension ring (CTR) with or without a suture. If the area of zonular loss is less than 3 clock hours, I would place a conventional CTR. If for some reason a CTR was not available, the IOL will usually remain in position in the sulcus with 3 clock hours or less of zonular dialysis. If the area of zonular loss is greater than 3 clock hours, I would suture a modified CTR (Cionni). If not available, I would be very cautious placing the IOL in a sulcus with this amount of zonular loss. I would try to place the IOL in the sulcus but have a very low threshold for iris suture fixation.

References

1. Amino K, Yamakawa R. Long-term results of out-of-the-bag intraocular lens implantation. *J Cataract Refract Surg.* 2000;26(2):266-270.
2. Oetting TA. Cataract Surgery for Greenhorns. MedRounds Publishing; 2005. Available at: http://www.medrounds.org/cataract-surgery-greenhorns. Accessed November 20, 2006.
3. Micheli T, Cheung LM, Sharma S, et al. Acute haptic-induced pigmentary glaucoma with an AcrySof intraocular lens. *J Cataract Refract Surg.* 2002;28(10):1869-1872.
4. LeBoyer RM, L Werner, Snyder ME, et al. Acute haptic-induced ciliary sulcus irritation associated with single-piece AcrySof intraocular lenses. *J Cataract Refract Surg.* 2005;31(7):1421-1427.
5. Maassen, J, Oetting T, Omphroy L. A constant for sulcus based MA60BM. Unpublished data presented at: University of Iowa Ophthalmology Resident Research Conference; Iowa City Iowa, May 19 2006. Available at http://webeye.ophth.uiowa.edu/dept/RESFELO/ResDay2006/abstracts/maassen.htm. Accessed Jan 3 2007.
6. Suto C, Hori S, Fukuyama E, Akura J. Adjusting intraocular lens power for sulcus fixation. *J Cataract Refract Surg.* 2003;29(10):1913-1917.

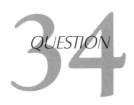

QUESTION

34

WHEN AND HOW SHOULD I SUTURE FIXATE A POSTERIOR CHAMBER INTRAOCULAR LENS?

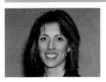

Elizabeth A. Davis, MD, FACS

Most cataract surgery performed today in the United States is extracapsular cataract extraction (ECCE) phacoemulsification with implantation of a posterior chamber intraocular lens (PCIOL). When an intact posterior capsule is present, almost all surgeons favor in-the-bag placement of a PCIOL. However, in the absence of capsular support, the type of implant to place and the technique used to secure the implant in the eye are much more controversial.

Anterior chamber intraocular lenses (ACIOLs) are the easiest to insert, but they have been associated with various complications, including pseudophakic bullous keratopathy, iris atrophy, glaucoma, and the uveitis-glaucoma-hyphema syndrome. Nevertheless, the newer Kelman multiflex style, open-loop AC lenses are a significant improvement over the previous closed-loop lenses. However, these lenses cannot be used without adequate iris support or when there is significant angle pathology.

Sutured PCIOLs move the implant away from the corneal endothelium and anterior chamber angle and closer to the nodal point of the eye. They are thus less likely to cause endothelial cell loss, peripheral anterior synechiae, or secondary angle-closure glaucoma. Two options exist for posterior chamber IOL suture fixation: iris or transscleral fixation.

Iris Fixation

McCannel[1] described fixation of the haptics of a PCIOL to the iris in 1976. This method (Figure 34-1) is performed by inserting the haptics of the PCIOL into the ciliary sulcus and

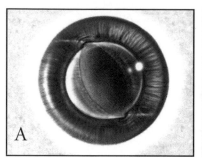
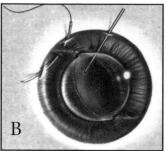
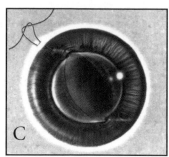
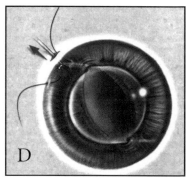
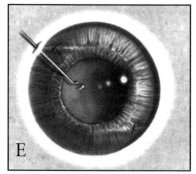

Figure 34-1. (A) The optic is captured with the pupil. (B) The suture is passed through the peripheral cornea, through the iris, under the haptic, back up through the iris, and out the peripheral cornea. (C) The sutures are pulled through a paracentesis with a hook. (D) A knot is tied and the suture ends are cut. (E) The optic is repositioned posterior to the iris. (Reprinted from *Intraocular Lenses in Cataract and Refractive Surgery*, Azar DT, ed, Ashraf MF, Stark WJ, McCannel sutures and secondary iris-fixated intraocular lenses, 166-167, © 2001, with permission from Elsevier.)

capturing the optic by the pupil, generally with the help of a miotic agent like Miochol (Novartis Pharmaceuticals, East Hanover, NJ). A 9-0 or 10-0 polypropylene suture on a long needle such as a CIF-4 (Ethicon Inc, Sommerville, NJ) or PC-7 (Alcon Laboratories, Fort Worth, Tex) is then passed through the peripheral cornea, through the iris, beneath the haptic, up through the iris, and back out through the peripheral cornea. The suture ends are then pulled through a paracentesis with a Kuglen (Katena Eye Instruments, Denville, NJ) or Sinskey (Bausch & Lomb Storz, San Dimas, Calif) hook and tied, cinching the knot down onto the iris. Once both haptics are fixated, the optic is prolapsed posteriorly behind the iris.

In 2004, Chang[2] described the use of a Siepser sliding knot for this technique. This method avoids excessive iris traction but requires either the use of microscissors or a large enough incision to allow insertion of Vannas scissors.

Iris fixation has the benefits of being faster and perhaps easier than transscleral fixation. Furthermore, one is working through a closed system that minimizes the risk of intraoperative hypotony (and its attendant risk of choroidal hemorrhage) and infectious complications. However, there is a much greater chance of pupil distortion. Lens decentration, optic tilt, uveitis, pigment dispersion, and hyphema can also rarely occur.

Transscleral Fixation

For transscleral fixation, there are several variations of each step of this technique; it would be far too extensive to describe all of them here. Por and Lavin have described a complete, detailed review of these methods.[3] I will, however, outline the major steps of the procedure.

To begin, the surgeon must select a lens. Although square knots or slipknots can be used to fixate almost any PCIOL, special haptic designs have been created for transscleral fixation. Haptics with enlarged ends (either premanufactured or created by the surgeon with cautery) prevent knot slippage. Additionally, holes or eyelets in the haptics allow passage of suture at equidistances from the optic on either side.

Prior to suturing a PCIOL transsclerally, it is important to perform a thorough vitrectomy. This prevents vitreous from displacing the IOL or prolapsing around the edges of the optic. Furthermore, incarceration of vitreous with the sutures can cause traction on the retina and potentially lead to a retinal detachment. I prefer to use a large (6.5 mm to 7.0 mm) optic for these cases. The large optic is a little more forgiving than a smaller one in case of any decentration.

The introduction of sutures can be done via an ab externo (from the outside in) or an ab interno (from the inside out) approach. The ab interno procedure is faster, but it is also a blind procedure. The ab externo procedure, though technically more challenging, allows greater accuracy in suture placement.

Securing the haptic with the suture can be done with square knots, slip knots, or girth hitches. When eyelets are present, sutures can be passed through them for 2-, 3-, or 4-point fixation. A greater number of fixation points have less risk of inducing tilt or decentration but also require great care to avoid entangling multiple sutures.

Sutures may exit vertically or obliquely, but a 3:00 and 9:00 exit should be avoided to prevent encountering the ciliary vessels. Radial keratotomy markers can be used to facilitate placing diametrically opposed fixation points. Knowledge of the location of the ciliary sulcus (0.83 mm and 0.46 mm posterior to the limbus in the vertical and horizontal meridians, respectively) is also important for proper suture placement.

Knots should be buried in the sclera and covered with conjunctiva or alternatively covered with scleral flaps.

Although excellent results have been achieved with transsclerally sutured PCIOLs, complications are not rare. The sutures may erode through the scleral flaps and cause irritation. Additionally, they may loosen or break and cause tilting or dislocation of the optic. A persistent suture extending between intraocular and extraocular environments may provide a tract for bacteria to enter the eye and establish endophthalmitis. Choroidal hemorrhage and detachment can occur from inadvertent injury to the ciliary body. Traction on the peripheral retina or vitreous during suture placement in the sulcus may increase the risk of retinal detachment. It is interesting to note that despite uncomplicated placement of these polypropylene sutures, histopathologic studies have shown that the distal haptics probably lie outside the ciliary sulcus. Some authors have advocated using an endoscope to confirm placement of sulcus sutures.

Late cases of sutured IOL dislocations have been reported. In our own experience of over 15 years at Minnesota Eye Consultants, we are aware of 8 patients who have had suture erosion and lens dislocation of implants that were transsclerally sutured an average of 10 years prior. All required surgical repair, which was quite challenging in certain cases. Because of reports and experience with cases such as these, some surgeons advocate use of 9-0 rather than 10-0 polypropylene or even 8-0 Gore-tex suture.

Despite these rare but significant late complications, suturing of PCIOLs plays a role in cases of capsular compromise. They are preferred to ACIOLs when the cornea shows signs of compromise (eg, guttatae), if the anterior chamber is shallow, or if the patient has glaucoma or angle pathology. Each case is unique and the surgical management must be individualized.

References

1. McCannel MA. A retrievable suture idea for anterior uveal problems. *Ophthalmic Surg.* 1976;7:98-103.
2. Chang DF. Siepser slipknot for McCannel iris-suture fixation of subluxated intraocular lenses. *J Cataract Refract Surg.* 2004;30:1170-1176.
3. Por YM, Lavin MJ. Techniques or intraocular lens suspension in the absence of capsular/zonular support. *Surv Ophthalmol.* 2005;50:429-462.

35

WHEN AND HOW SHOULD I IMPLANT AN ANTERIOR CHAMBER (ANGLE-SUPPORTED) INTRAOCULAR LENS?

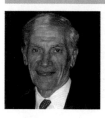

Manus C. Kraff, MD

Life is cyclical, and intraocular lenses (IOLs) appear to be also. Historically, angle-supported (mistakenly called anterior chamber) IOLs* (AS IOLs) date back to the early 1950s with the lenses of Danheim, Strampelli, and Barraquer. These lenses caused a great deal of problems because of the materials used, design, and manufacturing techniques. Because of these problems, AS lenses are used in 1.5% of IOL implantations today. This is about to change, but it is still appropriate to discuss the current indications for use of AS lenses and their future (Figure 35-1).

The current indications for AS IOLs are as follows:

* Secondary implantation (after a current or previous intracapsular cataract extraction)

* Rupture of the posterior capsule during cataract surgery with insufficient capsular support for a posterior chamber (PC) IOL[1]

* After removal of a subluxated PC IOL with insufficient capsular support remaining (Figure 35-2)

Suturing of PC IOLs is currently being performed when inadequate capsular support exists for implantation of a posterior chamber IOL. In my opinion, an AS lens is a far better choice for both the patient and the surgeon. This is because an AS IOL is technically

---

* Angle-supported lenses are one form of anterior chamber lenses in addition to iris-supported lenses such as the "lobster claw" and the "Verisyse." The author feels anterior chamber IOL (ACIOL) is really only a half truth and therefore wants to present an accurate description (AS) and name.

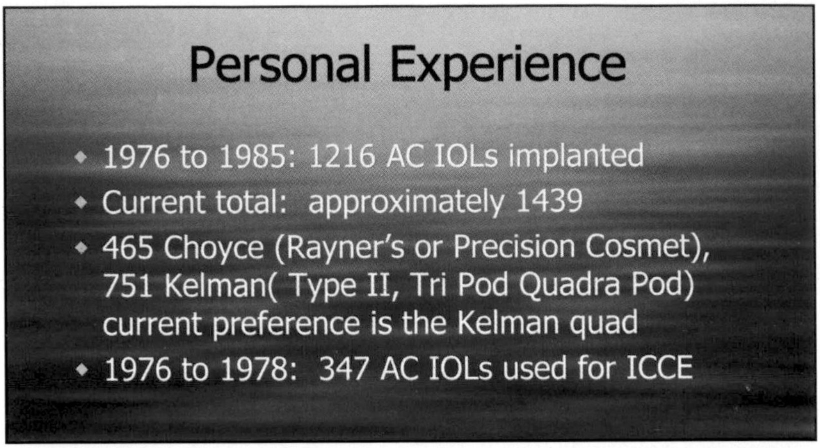

Figure 35-1. Current indications for use of AS lenses and their future.

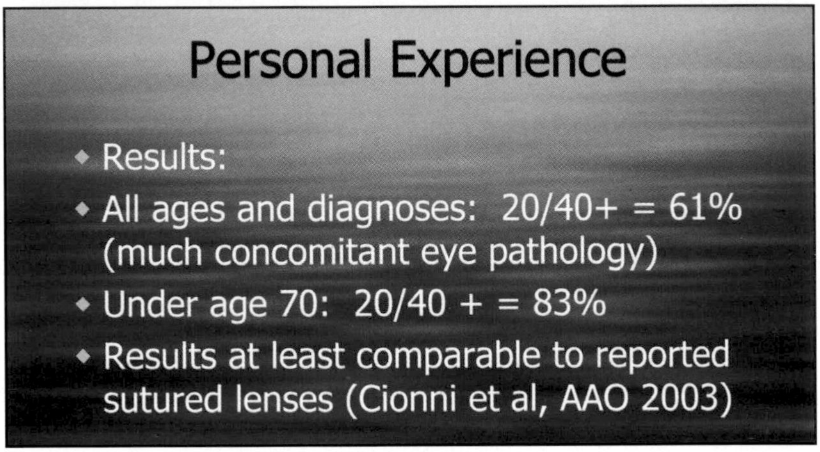

Personal Experience

- 1976 to 1985: 1216 AC IOLs implanted
- Current total: approximately 1439
- 465 Choyce (Rayner's or Precision Cosmet), 751 Kelman(Type II, Tri Pod Quadra Pod) current preference is the Kelman quad
- 1976 to 1978: 347 AC IOLs used for ICCE

Figure 35-2. Current indication for use of AS lenses includes after removal of a subluxated posterior chamber (PC) IOL with insufficient capsular support remaining.

Personal Experience

- Results:
- All ages and diagnoses: 20/40+ = 61% (much concomitant eye pathology)
- Under age 70: 20/40 + = 83%
- Results at least comparable to reported sutured lenses (Cionni et al, AAO 2003)

much easier to implant, less surgical time is required for the procedure, and the implantation of an AS IOL is far less traumatic to the eye then suturing a PC IOL. The AS lens is far easier to remove if indicated than a sutured PC IOL (Figure 35-3). The AS lenses are in contact with the anterior surface of the iris, which is derived from mesodermal tissue as contrasted to a sutured posterior chamber IOL, which is in contact with the iris pigment layer, which is derived from neural ectoderm, which causes much more intraocular inflammation and cystoid macular edema in the postsurgical period, and also has a far greater incidence of late hemorrhaging into the anterior chamber.

Sizing of these lenses is still determined by measuring the white-to-white distance under a microscope with a caliper. This is about to change with the newer anterior segment-imaging devices such as the Visante OCT (Carl Zeiss Meditec, Jena, Germany), the Oculus Pentacam (Lynwood, Wash), and the Artemis VHF digital ultrasound scanner (Ultralink LLC, St. Petersburg, Fla).

In a review of my own data with more than 1500 AS IOLs over a 25-year period, the results are superior to sutured PC IOLs.

Insertion of the AS lens is through a 6-mm limbal incision, usually temporally, on top of a Sheets glide. The incision is closed with 2 or 3 interrupted 10-0 nylon sutures. At least one surgical peripheral iridectomy is required to prevent postoperative papillary block.

Personal Experience

* Review of angle-supported IOLs implanted in the last 10 years: 108 lenses = 1% to 1.5% of total lenses implanted (Alcon noted similar 1% of AC IOL sales)
* Secondary IOL: Post previous ICCE = 40%
* Removal and replacement of AC or PC IOL and post PKP = 30%
* Inadequate capsular support = 19%
* ICCE = 11% (primary surgery)

Figure 35-3. An AS lens is far easier to remove if indicated than a sutured PC IOL.

This is accomplished by a small limbal incision superior to the temporal wound with pressure on the posterior lip. If the iris does not prolapse spontaneously, one may extract it with a fine tooth forceps and perform the iridectomy.

You should not place a posterior chamber lens in the anterior chamber because you will encounter all of the problems of the poorly designed AS lens era (ie, "cocooning" of the haptics in the angle with resultant inflammation, cystoid macular edema, glaucoma, and the necessity for late lens removal). As we have learned, lenses must be flexible and have flat footplates at the periphery of the haptics.

Another important reason for developing a familiarity with AS IOLs is that I think the cycle is continuing. In the not-too-distant future, an AS IOL will be used for the correction of phakic refractive errors.

In my opinion, within 10 years, AS phakic IOLs will be the refractive procedure of choice. You ask "why?"

Currently, there are US and European companies with ongoing clinical trials involving AS phakic IOLs. These lenses will be very easy to implant. The procedure will be reversible and may be explanted easily if necessary. They will fold into a cartridge and be injected into the anterior chamber through a very small wound that is astigmatically neutral. The ease of the procedure will enable almost all ophthalmologists to perform implantation of these lenses. They have superior design features to the currently available AS IOLs. All European studies have shown that lenticular correction of refractive errors is optically superior to a corneal procedure in refractive surgery. Visual return will be almost immediate, producing patient satisfaction.

Yes, the cycle continues.

References

1. Kwong YY, Yuen HK, Lam RF, Lee VY, Rao SK, Lam DS. Comparison of outcomes of primary scleral-fixated versus primary anterior chamber intraocular lens implantation in complicated cataract surgeries. *Ophthalmology.* 2007;114(1):80-85. Epub 2006 Oct 27.

QUESTION 36

BASED UPON THE ESCRS RANDOMIZED STUDY, SHOULD I USE INTRACAMERAL ANTIBIOTICS? WHICH AGENT?

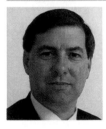

Eric D. Donnenfeld, MD

Cataract surgery is one of the most commonly performed operations in the United States, with approximately 3 million procedures performed annually.[1] Modern cataract surgery has become a safe and minimally invasive procedure that continues to produce excellent outcomes. Although the incidence of endophthalmitis is extremely low, the large volume of cataract surgeries produces approximately 4000 cases of endophthalmitis per year (Figure 36-1), with potentially devastating consequences.

The basic principles of antibiotic prophylaxis are as follows:

* To deliver an active agent effective against infecting micro-organisms
* To have adequate contact time between the drug and the infecting microbe since most antibiotics require bacterial replication to completely kill of the organism
* To avoid or minimize toxicity and side effects
* To minimize the risk of developing antibiotic-resistant organisms
* To be affordable

Antibiotic prophylaxis for the prevention of endophthalmitis in cataract surgery is one of the most controversial areas in ophthalmology. This is due to the ocular morbidity of

Figure 36-1. Endophthalmitis following cataract surgery.

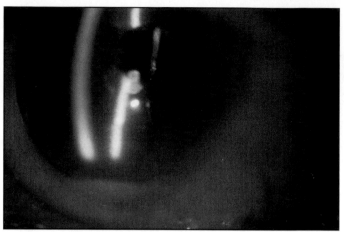

endophthalmitis coupled with the paucity of clinical studies that conclusively show an effective technique to reduce its occurrence.

Intrinsically, the concept of placing an antibiotic into the target tissue of the anterior chamber to eradicate or partially treat the potential bacterial inoculum that occurs at the time of surgery makes sense. A number of retrospective studies have suggested that intracameral antibiotics can significantly reduce the risk of ocular infection. In the 1990s, for instance, no cases of endophthalmitis occurred in a large series of cataract surgeries where gentamicin and vancomycin were placed in the irrigation bottle.[2] Today, a significant number of surgeons are using intracameral antibiotics during cataract surgery. Intracameral antibiotics can either be placed into the irrigating bottle or can be directly injected into the eye at the conclusion of the case. While placing the antibiotic into the infusion fluid may be simpler, I prefer to inject the antibiotic into the anterior chamber using a separate syringe after intraocular lens implantation. This allows me to achieve a high and reproducible concentration. This also reduces the toxicity risk of an overdose of intracameral antibiotic, which theoretically could occur from excessive irrigation volumes during prolonged surgical cases.

The most common intracameral antibiotics used today are vancomycin and tobramycin. However, these antibiotics may not be the ideal intraocular agents. Both vancomycin and tobramycin are relatively toxic and only low concentrations may be safely employed. The aminoglycosides are toxic to the retina, and clinicians have documented macula infarction following the inadvertent intracameral injection of undiluted tobramycin. Vancomycin may be associated with cystoid macular edema following cataract surgery.[3] Due to the low concentrations employed and the rapid turnover of aqueous humor, there may be insufficient levels of vancomycin and tobramycin to effectively kill organisms inside the eye. The limited gram-positive spectrum coverage with the aminoglycosides and minimal gram negative coverage with vancomycin are also of concern. Moreover, vancomycin is not the ideal intracameral agent because it is an extremely slow-acting bactericidal antibiotic. The Centers for Disease Control and Prevention has recommended that vancomycin not be used for prophylaxis in cataract surgery.

The ESCRS endophthalmitis prophylaxis study is the latest and by far the most important study to document the importance of intracameral antibiotics, specifically intracameral cefuroxime, in preventing endophthalmitis. It is the first prospective, controlled, double-masked, multicenter study to look at this issue.[4] In this study, there was a 5-fold reduction in endophthalmitis in patients receiving cefuroxime as compared to patients who did not receive any intracameral antibiotic. However, another important question that emerges from this study is exactly what is the best antibiotic to use intracamerally? Cefuroxime may not be used in patients with penicillin allergy and has limited gram-negative coverage. The ideal intracameral antibiotic would be broad spectrum, bactericidal, fast acting, nontoxic, and could be supplemented with topical dosing.

Fourth-generation fluoroquinolones are concentration-dependent killers in that they must reach the minimal inhibitory concentrations (MICs) in order to be effective. Recent studies evaluating MICs have shown that this class of agents appears to cover bacteria resistant to the second- and third-generation fluoroquinolones and is significantly more potent against gram-positive and gram-negative bacteria. The fourth-generation fluoroquinolones offer several major theoretical advantages over previously employed intracameral antibiotics. Gatifloxacin and moxifloxacin, for example, have rapid bactericidal action, steep kill curves,[5] and high solubility and may be absorbed into intraocular tissues to provide a more sustained release. They are less toxic to the cornea and retina, provide excellent gram-positive and gram-negative coverage, and can be supplemented by the topical administration of commercially available gatifloxacin (Zymar, Allergan, Inc, Irvine, Calif) and moxifloxacin (Vigamox, Alcon Laboratories, Inc, Fort Worth, Tex) to prolong their therapeutic aqueous concentration. In a rabbit model, Snyder et al showed that as much as 320 µg of gatifloxacin in the anterior chamber is well tolerated, with no sign of corneal clouding, glaucoma, or retinal toxicity.[6]

We used intracameral gatifloxacin in a single eye of 40 patients following routine cataract surgery with clear corneal incisions.[7] All patients received 100 µg of the IV solution diluted in balanced salt solution (BSS) into 0.1 mL, which was injected into the middle of the anterior chamber (see Formulating Intracameral Cefuroxime below). In all cases, the eyes tolerated the antibiotic well and displayed no signs of corneal or retinal toxicity. This intracameral dose should maintain therapeutic levels 5 times longer than the same concentration of vancomycin that ophthalmologists most commonly use.

The ideal intracameral antibiotic would be broad spectrum, bactericidal, fast acting, nontoxic, and able to be supplemented with topical medications. Directly injecting intracameral antibiotic at the conclusion of surgery ensures that the dosage is both sufficient and nontoxic (toxicity can occur when the antibiotic is placed in the irrigating solution during a complex cataract extraction). In my experience, intracameral gatifloxacin appears safe in human eyes at a dosage of 100 µg in 0.1 mL. Studies are also underway to investigate the use of intracameral moxifloxacin. For now, however, based on the peer review literature, I recommend intracameral cefuroxime until controlled, masked studies have been performed with the fluoroquinolones.

Formulating Intracameral Cefuroxime

Intracameral cefuroxime is formulated by taking the IV formulation of 750 mg cefuroxime in 50 mL and diluting it with 25 mL of BSS, which results in 750 mg of cefuroxime in 75 mL or 10 mg/mL. This solution is then filtered under sterile conditions using a

0.2-mm filter. A sterile, 26-gauge irrigating cannula is attached to a sterile tuberculin syringe and 1 mg of cefuroxime in 0.1 mL is injected through the paracentesis into the center of the anterior chamber. The solution is mixed daily and used for a full day's schedule of surgeries.

References

1. Javitt JC, Kendix M, Tielsch JM, et al. Geographical variation in utilization of cataract surgery. *Med Care.* 1995;33:90-105.
2. Gimbel HV, Sun R, DeBroff BM. Prophylactic intracameral antibiotics during cataract surgery: the incidence of endophthalmitis and corneal endothelial loss. *Eur J Implant Refract Surg.* 1994;6:280-285.
3. Blumenthal M. Prophylactic intracameral vancomycin and CME. *Ophthalmology.* 2000;107:1616-1617.
4. Barry P, Seal DV, Gettinby G, et al. ESCRS study of prophylaxis of postoperative endophthalmitis after cataract surgery: preliminary report of principal results from a European multicenter study. *J Cataract Refract Surg.* 2006;32:407-410.
5. Mather R, Karenchak LM, Romanowski EG, Kowalski RP. Fourth-generation fluoroquinolones: new weapons in the arsenal of ophthalmic antibiotics. *Am J Ophthalmol.* 2002;133(4):463-466.
6. Snyder RW, Chang M, Hare W, et al. Intraocular safety of gatifloxacin in a rabbit model. Paper presented at: The Ocular Microbiology and Immunology Group Meeting; November 15, 2003; Anaheim, Calif.
7. Donnenfeld ED, Snyder RW, Kanellopolous AJ, et al. Safety of prophylactic intracameral gatifloxacin in cataract surgery. Paper presented at: The Ocular Microbiology and Immunology Group Meeting; November 15, 2003; Anaheim, Calif.

WHEN DO YOU USE INTRACAMERAL DRUGS (AND AT WHAT DOSAGES) FOR CATARACT SURGERY?

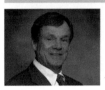

James P. Gills, MD

Improving cataract surgery outcomes and minimizing recovery are keys to satisfied patients and a successful practice. Intracameral medications are one method for making cataract surgery simpler and safer and are a focus of a great deal of my time and energy. Over the years I have developed techniques for using intracameral anesthesia, antibiotics, anti-inflammatories, and, most recently, investigating antivascular endothelial growth factor (VEGF) medications for my cataract patients. There are 5 reasons that explain why I feel so strongly about the importance of intraocular medications with cataract surgery and I call them the 5 Cs:

1. Compliance: Only 37% of patients are totally compliant with their medications.

2. Convenience: Patients and doctors want the simplest postoperative regimen with the fewest medications as possible.

3. Cost: Intracameral prepared medications cost one-third the price of prescribed topical medications. The cost of medications is shifting from the patient to the surgeon and surgical facility.

4. Comfort: Eliminates the problems associated with topical medications. The toxic effects of preservatives on the cornea are eliminated.

5. Control: Administering intraocular medications gives the patient a controlled dosage and placement at the site.

Table 37-1

Protocol for Topical/Intraocular Anesthesia

Preoperative

Alcaine 0.5% (Alcon Laboratories, Inc)	1 to 2 gtt x 1
Mydriacyl 0.5% (Alcon Laboratories, Inc)	1 to 2 gtt x 1
Buffered Betadine (Purdue Pharma LP, Stamford, Conn)/BSS	1 to 2 gtt x 1
Dilating gel	1 gtt in the operative eye every 5 minutes x 2

5 cc viscous Xylocaine 2% (AstraZeneca LP, Coral Gables, Fla)
1 cc NeoSynephrine 10% (Neofrin) (Cynacon/OCuSOFT Inc, Rosenberg, Tex)
1 cc Mydriacyl 1%
2 cc Zymar
1 cc Acular (Allergan, Inc, Irvine, Calif)

Operating Room

Alcaine 0.5%	1 gtt x 1 OU
Buffered Betadine/BSS	1 gtt x 3 (2 gtts at the beginning of the case, the 3rd gtt at the end of the case)

Preparation: Draw up 20 cc BSS followed by 1 cc of Betadine solution 10%. Add 1.4 cc Na Bicarb 8.4%. Change needle to 18-gauge filter needle and inject into sterile dropperette. Zymar 1 gtt postop in the operative eye.

Intraocular Xylocaine 1% preservative free, without epinephrine

Preparation: To 15 cc BSS add 3.75 mL sodium bicarbonate. Withdraw 15 mL of the buffered solution; mix with 5 mL of Xylocaine MPF 4%. This will yield a Xylocaine 1% buffered solution. 0.25 cc is used prophylactically after the incision is made to minimize patient discomfort.

Irrigation Solution

Epinephrine 1:1000
Ascorbic acid 1.76 mg/mL
500-mL bottle BSS
 Preparation:
To 500 mL bottle BSS add:
        0.5 mL epinephrine (1:1000)
        1.76 cc ascorbic acid (500 mg/mL)

A 0.22-μm micropore filter is used to filter all irrigation solutions.

Anesthesia

I integrated the use of intracameral preservative-free 1% lidocaine into my anesthesia regimen in 1994. The injection before the placement of viscoelastic provides a more pleasant surgical experience for both the patient and physician because it eliminates all sensation, including pressure.[1] Intraocular lidocaine is safe; however, toxicity and toxic anterior segment syndrome can be caused by high doses of many medications. We use 0.3 cc and make sure it is in the eye for a short time (Table 37-1).

Antibiotics

Thirty-three years ago, we started using intraocular antibiotics and filtering the irrigating solutions following several cases of sterile endophthalmitis associated with the implants. Over the last 30 years, we have changed from administering vancomycin in the irrigation bottle to injecting it intracamerally. This provides the patient with a controlled dosage at the desired location.

For my antibiotic regimen, I currently inject a total of 0.1 cc of BSS containing 33.3 mcg of vancomycin and 20 mcg of ceftazidime, along with dexamethasone (Table 37-2). While the idea of antibiotic prophylaxis has been surrounded by controversy, the possibility of creating resistance in the "closed container" of the globe is remote. My infection rate using the protocol I have described is less than 1 in 20,000 cases, and I attribute that primarily to my intraocular antibiotic regimen and the use of the Surgeon absolute 0.22-μm filter[2].

Anti-Inflammatories

To minimize inflammation, we have used various medications in the intracameral injection mixture, including dexamethasone (200 mcg to 400 mcg) and Kenalog (0.5 mg to 4 mg) (Bristol-Myers Squibb Co, New York, NY). I have found that Kenalog increases the pressure in about 6% of patients if more than 2 mg is administered. However, it can actually lower the pressure if less than 1.5 mg is given (Figures 37-1 and 37-2). The disadvantage of administering Kenalog at the time of surgery is that you lose the "wow" effect in the early postop period. Table 37-3 shows how to prepare a postoperative injection that delivers Kenalog 10 mg/1 cc AC solution. Up to 0.5 cc of Kenalog can be used without a high incidence of secondary glaucoma. I have found that 0.3 cc of Kenalog 20 mg is an ideal adjunct to the anti-inflammatory medications and has few side effects.

I pretreat patients with significant macular disease or diabetic retinopathy with one or more intravitreal injections of Avastin (Genetech, San Francisco, Calif) and Kenalog 1 week prior to surgery. I have also found that preoperative administration of anti-VEGF decreases the need for postoperative drops. I order optical coherence tomography (OCT) on all patients with retinal disease preoperatively, as suggested by Carmen Puliafito, MD. I have come to rely on OCT to monitor the patients' progress. Using this technology has tremendously improved our ability to detect and treat retinal disease. We are now able to help patients with retinal disease that we previously were not able to help before. I also include Kenalog in the postoperative injection to further reduce the risk of inflammation. Interestingly, no additional topical drops are needed in cases in which both Kenalog and Avastin are used.

Using medication intracamerally has always been somewhat controversial. The debate over the use of intracameral antibiotics because of the concern over resistant organisms is more academic than practical. It is far more likely to develop resistance with topical antibiotic prophylaxis than by administering antibiotics into a closed, sterile container. Since both the organism and the antibiotic are in a closed container, neither can spread. A 2005 multicenter ESCRS study of nearly 14,000 patients showed that those who did not receive intraocular antibiotics were 5 times more likely to develop endophthalmitis.[3] I have seen

---

Table 37-2

Postoperative Anterior Chamber Antibiotic/Anti-Inflammatory Injection

List of Supplies

1	BSS	500 mL
1	Vancomycin hydrochloride injection 500 mg	50 mg/mL
1	Ceftazidime 1 g	50 mg/mL
1	Dexamethasone	4 mg/mL
2	20-cc syringe	
1	5-cc syringe	
1	20 cc sterile water	
3	Tuberculin (TB) syringes	
1	Sterile empty vial	20 mL
6	5-µm filter needle	
7	20-gauge needles	

Reconstitution of Medications

Vancomycin—Using the filter needle and a 10-cc syringe, withdraw 10-cc sterile water. Change to a 20-gauge needle and inject 10-cc sterile water into 500-mg vial of vancomycin. Solution expires in 1 week.

Ceftazidime—Vent the bottle using a 20-gauge needle. Use a filter needle to withdraw 20-cc BSS from the 500-cc bottle. Switch to a 20-gauge needle and add to the bottle of ceftazidime, leaving the 20-gauge "vent" needle in place. The solution expires in 1 week.

Directions for Mixing the AC Solution

Using the 5-µm filter needle, withdraw 11.01 cc of BSS into a 20-cc syringe from a 500-cc bottle of BSS. Switch to a 20-gauge needle, inject the BSS into an empty 20-cc vial. Using a 5-µm filter needle and a TB syringe, withdraw 11.25 cc of dexamethasone. Change to a 20-gauge needle and inject into the same sterile vial containing the BSS. Using a 5-µm filter needle and a TB syringe, withdraw 0.09 cc of ceftazidime. Change to a 20-gauge needle and inject into the same sterile vial. Using a 5-µm filter needle and a TB syringe, withdraw 0.15 cc of vancomycin. Change to a 20-gauge needle and inject into the same sterile vial. (Total volume is equal to 22.5 cc.)

The solution contains the following in 0.1 cc:
- Ceftazidime 20 mcg
- Vancomycin 33.3 mcg
- Dexamethasone 200 mcg

---

no evidence of retinal toxicity since implementing intracameral antibiotics more than 30 years ago.

The use of Kenalog during cataract surgery may also be scrutinized. As I have mentioned, one concern is the issue of pressure rise following the injection. It is true that when doses of more than 1.5 mg are used, the risk of elevated pressure increases. However, when used in appropriate doses, this is rarely a problem. There have been some reports of sterile endophthalmitis.[4,5] However, while the risk of this is low, we have taken the precaution of changing to preservative-free Kenalog, which we obtain from a

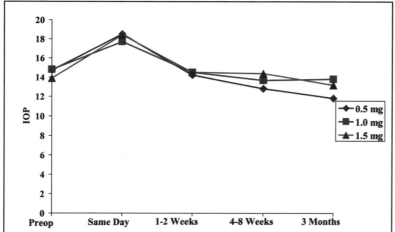

Figure 37-1. Mean intraocular pressure (IOP) over time.

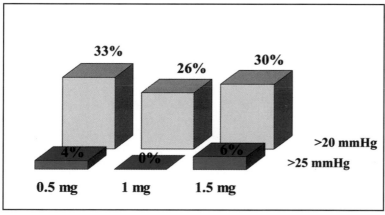

Figure 37-2. IOP spikes same day postoperatively.

compounding pharmacy. I believe the use of preservative-free Kenalog, along with Avastin, is an extremely effective tool in treating patients who are at risk for macular edema following cataract surgery and results in a quieter, safer postoperative course.

When properly used, intracameral medications improve the safety, cost effectiveness, convenience and reduce many complications such as macular edema, corneal edema, and keratitis. The future is very promising as we discover long-acting nonsteroidals, as well as new applications and ways to administer anti-VEGF drugs.

References

1. Gills JP, Cherchio MN, Raanan MG. Unpreserved lidocaine to control discomfort during cataract surgery using topical anesthesia. *J Cataract Refract Surg.* 1997;23(4):545-550.
2. Gills JP. Prevention of endophthalmitis by intraocular solution filtration and antibiotics. *J Am Intraocul Implant Soc.* 1985;11(2):185-186.
3. Barry P, Seal DV, Gettinby G, et al. ESCRS study of prophylaxis of postoperative endophthalmitis after cataract surgery: preliminary report of principal results from a European multicenter study. *J Cataract Refract Surg.* 2006;32(5):407-410.

Table 37-3

Postoperative Anterior Chamber
Antibiotic/Anti-inflammatory Injection With Kenalog

List of Supplies

1	BSS	500 mL
1	Vancomycin hydrochloride inj. 500 mg	50 mg/mL
1	Ceftazidime 1 GM	50 mg/mL
1	Dexamethasone	4 mg/mL
1	Kenalog	40 mg/mL
2	20-cc syringe	
1	5-cc syringe	
1	20-cc sterile water	
3	TB syringes	
1	Sterile empty vial	20 mL
6	5-µm filter needle	
8	20-gauge needles	

Reconstitution of Medications

Vancomycin—Using the filter needle and a 10-cc syringe, withdraw 10-cc sterile water. Change to a 20-gauge needle and inject 10-cc sterile water into a 500-mg vial of vancomycin. Solution expires in 1 week.

Ceftazidime—Vent the bottle using a 20-gauge needle. Use a filter needle to withdraw 20 cc of BSS from the 500-cc bottle. Switch to a 20-gauge needle and add to the bottle of ceftazidime, leaving the 20-gauge "vent" needle in place. Solution expires in 1 week.

Directions for Mixing the AC Solution

Using the 5-µm filter needle, withdraw 14.59 cc of BSS into a 20-cc syringe from a 500-cc bottle of BSS. Switch to a 20-gauge needle, inject the BSS into an empty 20-cc vial. Using a 5-µm filter needle and a TB syringe, withdraw 0.2 cc of dexamethasone. Change to a 20-gauge needle and inject into the same sterile vial containing the BSS. Using a 5-µm filter needle and a TB syringe, withdraw 0.08 cc of ceftazidime. Change to a 20-gauge needle and inject into the same sterile vial. Using a 5-µm filter needle and a TB syringe, withdraw 0.13 cc of vancomycin. Change to a 20-gauge needle and inject into the same sterile vial. Withdraw 5 cc of Kenalog using a 20-gauge needle and add to the same sterile vial. (Total volume is equal to 20 cc.)

Final Concentration

The Kenalog 10 mg/1 cc AC solution expires in 24 hours.

4. Kreissig I, Degenring RF, Jonas JB. Intravitreal triamcinolone acetonide complication of infectious and sterile endophthalmitis. *Ophthalmologe*. 2006;103(1):30-34.

5. Wang LC, Yang CM. Sterile endophthalmitis following intravitreal injection of triamcinolone acetonide. *Ocul Immunol Inflamm*. 2004;13(4):295-300.

SECTION III

POSTOPERATIVE QUESTIONS

WHAT IS THE BEST WAY TO PREVENT AND MANAGE POSTOPERATIVE INTRAOCULAR PRESSURE SPIKES?

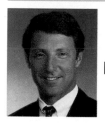

Richard A. Lewis, MD

Elevated intraocular pressure (IOP) is a common problem following cataract surgery. In some patients, this is a very transient problem while in others it can be vision threatening. Although it is not always predictable who will have a pressure rise, there is a group of patients at higher risk. In those patients, preventive measures instituted during surgery or immediately after the procedure are essential. Many patients can tolerate transient elevated IOP after cataract surgery; however, those with a history of glaucomatous cupping, compromised retinal vasculature, or corneal endothelial disease are vulnerable to complications especially when the IOP is over 30.

The most common reason for elevated IOP after uncomplicated cataract surgery is retained viscoelastic that blocks the egress of aqueous through the trabecular meshwork. This is a transient phenomenon that typically lasts 24 hours to 36 hours. However, the extent of the IOP elevation can be dramatic and concerning. This problem is best avoided by meticulous surgery with careful irrigation and aspiration of the viscoelastic material. Intracameral cholinergic agents appear to be of limited use in blunting the pressure rise caused by retained viscoelastic.

Postoperatively, there are various options to normalize the IOP in this setting (Table 38-1). The most direct approach involves releasing viscoelastic and aqueous from the eye (often referred to as "burping the wound") through the paracentesis site. This is performed in the exam room with the patient seated at the slit lamp. After checking the IOP (and with the eye topically anesthetized), I use a 30-gauge needle. I carefully penetrate the paracentesis site to allow a few drops of aqueous and viscoelastic to escape the wound. Gentle pressure with the needle on the posterior lip of the entry site facilitates release.

Table 38-1

Treatment for Elevated Pressure After Cataract Surgery

- Prophylaxis: remove viscoelastic at conclusion of surgery
- Paracentesis
- Medications
  - * Topical (Alpha agonist [ie, apraclonidine, beta blocker])
  - * Systemic (carbonic anhydrase inhibitor)

A speculum is usually unnecessary. Burping the wound can be repeated as needed to achieve an IOP at the desired level. I apply a topical antibiotic immediately afterward. It is important to remember that releasing aqueous through the paracentesis site may only reduce pressure for a brief time. Applying topical hypotensive drops helps maintain pressure reduction until the viscoelastic is completely gone.

Normalization of IOP after cataract surgery demands a fully functional outflow system. Patients with pre-existing ocular hypertension, glaucoma, or compromised outflow are at risk for a postoperative pressure rise. This may occur even following uncomplicated procedures because of surgical trauma and anterior segment inflammation. In these patients, it is useful to pre-treat with aqueous suppressants at the conclusion of surgery to prevent the pressure rise. I recommend using aqueous suppressants such as the alpha agonists (apraclonidine or brominidine), beta blockers (timolol), or carbonic anhydrase inhibitors (dorzolamide, brinzolamide, or oral acetazolamide). Sometimes a combination of these hypotensive agents may be necessary. Outflow drugs, such as the prostaglandin analogues in particular, are less effective in the immediate postoperative setting because they require a more prolonged onset of action and may induce anterior segment inflammation. In those patients with glaucomatous cupping and visual field loss, or any patient who can ill afford a marked postoperative pressure rise, combining cataract and glaucoma surgery may be recommended.

When considering the various causes of pressure elevation after cataract surgery, topical steroids are often suspected. However, steroids in the immediate postoperative period are rarely a cause of the pressure rise. Typically, a steroid-induced glaucoma requires 3 to 6 weeks of continuous dosing to elicit an IOP response. You should not see this in the immediate postoperative period.

Pressure problems should be anticipated in cataract patients following surgical complications, such as posterior capsular tears and vitreous loss with or without dropped lens fragments. The combination of prolonged surgery, inflammation, retained lens fragments, and modified intraocular lens placement should be a red flag for potential IOP problems. Careful clean-up of the anterior segment with removal of the residual lens material and prolapsing vitreous is important to avoid this problem (as well as other complications). Hypotensive medications following complicated cataract surgery are often ineffective at controlling IOP. Pars plana vitrectomy and lensectomy for a dropped nucleus and vitreous debris should be undertaken early in the postoperative period to control a persistently elevated pressure and to prevent other complications. Do not assume, however, that vitreous surgery alone will control the IOP for all such patients. Complicated cataract surgery impairs outflow facility and these patients can develop prolonged pressure elevation. Filtering surgery may be necessary for definitive pressure control.

Conclusion

IOP elevation after cataract surgery is not uncommon. Simple measures, including meticulous surgery, prophylactic medications in high-risk patients, and postoperative "burping" of a paracentesis, are useful measures to avoid pressure-related complications.

Bibliography

1. Fry LL. Comparison of the postoperative intraocular pressure with betagan betoptic, timoptic, iopidine, diamox, pilopine gel, and miostat. *J Cataract Refract Surg.* 1992;18:14-19.
2. Barak A, Desatnik H, Ma-Naim T, Ashkenazi I, Neufeld A, Melamed S. Early postoperative intraocular pressure pattern in glaucomatous and nonglaucomatous patients. *J Cataract Refract Surg.* 1996;22:607-611.
3. Rainer G, Menapace R, Schmetterer K, Findl O, Georgopoulos M, Vass C. Effect of dorzolamide and latanoprost on intraocular pressure after small incision cataract surgery. *J Cataract Refract Surg.* 1999;25:1624-1629.

ON POSTOPERATIVE DAY 1, THE ANTERIOR CHAMBER IS SHALLOW AND THE PATIENT IS UNEXPECTEDLY VERY MYOPIC. WHAT SHOULD I DO?

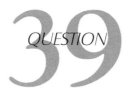

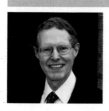

Luther L. Fry, MD

The differential diagnosis for this problem is relatively short and includes wound leak, choroidal hemorrhage or effusion, aqueous misdirection, and capsular block (Figure 39-1). A wound leak is by far the most likely cause of a shallow chamber.

A wound leak is relatively easy to detect. If the intraocular pressure (IOP) is near zero there is probably a wound leak. I use the Seidel test to confirm the leak. On the rare occasion where a wound leak is detected with a positive Seidel test, with either a shallow or normal depth anterior chamber, I usually take the patient back to the operating room and place an "X" suture (Figure 39-2). This is easily done under topical anesthesia and only takes a couple of minutes. The patient tends not to view this additional step as a complication or a "re-do." I use a full sterile set-up and drape, but I have in the past done this in the office minor surgical room with a lid speculum, gloves, and no drape.

With a formed anterior chamber and a wound leak, you could also consider either observing the patient or placing a bandage contact lens. These options would be useful if going back to the operating room is difficult such as when the operating room is in a hospital setting and a minor surgery room is not available in your office. However, in our surgicenter, placing a suture is almost as easy as placing a bandage contact lens. As mentioned above, the patient does not view it as a re-intervention. When we previously did surgery in the hospital, placing a suture was a major production, requiring re-admission, lots of patient anxiety, and extra expense. Suturing is certainly a more definitive

Figure 39-1. Differential diagnosis for shallow chamber and myopic shift.

Shallow Chamber and Myopic Shift 1 Day Postcataract Surgery

•Pressure low: ***Wound leak***, *check for Seidel Suture (preferred) or bandage lens*
•Pressure normal: ***Choroidal effusion*** *(or heme) Observe*
•Pressure high: ***Aqueous misdirection*** *Atropine; disrupt anterior hyaloid with YAG laser, needle aspiration, or pars plana vitrectomy*

Figure 39-2. "X" suture.

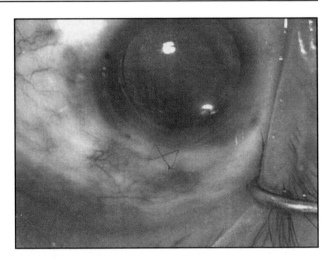

treatment and spares both the patient and the surgeon any further anxiety. This is my preference if it can be done easily. However, I think the risk of endophthalmitis in this setting is very low and a couple days of watchful waiting is reasonable.

If the chamber is shallow, the incision is Seidel negative, and the IOP is normal to slightly elevated, it is possible that a choroidal effusion or hemorrhage has occurred. Indirect ophthalmoscopy or B-scan ultrasound should demonstrate the presence of a choroidal effusion or hemorrhage. Watchful waiting and careful observation can suffice for smaller choroidals, but if the choroidal is large enough to cause a shallow chamber, drainage may be necessary. Choroidals will very rarely occur with uncomplicated small incision surgery. In my personal experience, choroidals following cataract surgery were more common with the large incision planned extra capsular surgery I did years ago, and fortunately they have become pretty much a thing of the past with modern small incision surgery.

Interestingly, I think wound leak in the first few minutes following surgery may be more common than we would like to think.[1,2] I recently did a study with 50 consecutive uncomplicated cataract surgeries where I measured IOP with a tonopen immediately after the speculum and drape were removed. Twenty-six percent (13 out of 50) of these patients had an IOP of 5 mm Hg or less. Prior to finishing the case I had filled the anterior chamber to a high pressure by tactile finger estimation, then I used my typical technique to express fluid through the side-port incision to what I estimated to be a mid-teens pressure. Interestingly, by 3 hours to 5 hours later when I did my same day check, none out of the 50 patients had an IOP less than 10, and 50% were above 25. (Yes, I do remove viscoelastic.) Although immediate wound leak may occur, it is likely in the living eye that these leaks quickly seal (so cadaver studies may need to be discounted with this disclaimer).

These transient wound leaks are, of course, a concern because they may increase the risk of postoperative bacterial endophthalmitis.[3] By being alert to possible wound leaks and suturing them promptly when they occurred, I have been fortunate to have had no cases of endophthalmitis for the past 5000 cataract operations.

If the chamber is shallow and the IOP is elevated, one may either have pupillary block or aqueous misdirection. Pupillary block with a posterior chamber intraocular lens (IOL) is very rare and I have not seen this despite not making an iridotomy in over 30,000 cases. Fortunately, I have also have had no personal experience with postcataract surgery aqueous misdirection. If confronted with this, I would probably first do a laser iridotomy. If the chamber did not immediately deepen, I would try to get through the peripheral capsule with the YAG back into the vitreous. If still not successful, I would open the posterior capsule and disrupt the anterior vitreous. If successful, I would keep the patient on atropine for a prolonged period of time. If not successful, I would refer the patient to a vitreoretinal surgeon for a core vitrectomy. If ready access to a vitreoretinal surgeon is not available, one might first try vitreous aspiration with a #20 or #22 needle through the pars plana.

Capsular block syndrome would also be a possible cause of a myopic shift due to a more forward location of the IOL optic. This may or may not be associated with shallowing of the anterior chamber. The most frequent cause is retained viscoelastic behind the IOL optic. The diagnosis should be obvious by observing the distended posterior capsule behind the IOL. I have also not personally seen this early on, although mild degrees are quite common several years postoperatively. Some cases of capsular block syndrome will resolve spontaneously. A peripheral YAG opening in the anterior capsule can allow enough trapped fluid to exit the capsular bag to allow the IOL to move posteriorly. Finally, removing the retained viscoelastic in the operating room remains a last resort if other measures fail.

Late capsular block syndrome, noted incidentally when the patient comes in for his or her YAG laser capsulotomy several years after surgery, is common. It is obvious at slit lamp, with the distended space between the IOL and posterior capsule filled with turbid fluid. It goes away immediately after YAG laser capsulotomy and is not associated with any excessive iritis post-YAG. Late capsular block syndrome is not usually associated with any shallowing of the anterior chamber or refractive power changes.

Immediate postoperative hypotony and shallow chamber with the accompanying myopic shift are aggravating; however, they need not be disastrous. For leaking incisions, immediate suturing under topical anesthesia, or careful monitoring, possibly after placement of a bandage contact lens, can rescue these rare situations without permanent damage to anything but the surgeon's coronaries.

References

1. Fry EL. Immediate postoperative intraocular pressures after routine topical clear corneal cataract surgery. Free paper presented at: ASCRS Symposium; March 19, 2006.
2. Taban M, Sarayba MA, Ignacio TS, et al. Ingress of India ink into the anterior chamber through sutureless clear corneal cataract wounds. *Arch Ophthalmol.* 2005;123:643-648.
3. Nagaki Y, Hayasaka S, Kadoi C, et al. Bacterial endophthalmitis after small-incision cataract surgery. *J Cataract Refract Surg.* 2003;29:20-26.

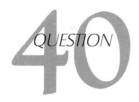

QUESTION

40

FOLLOWING UNEVENTFUL SURGERY, THREE OF MY EIGHT PATIENTS HAVE 4+ CELL AND FIBRIN ON POSTOPERATIVE DAY 1. WHAT SHOULD I DO?

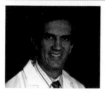

Nick Mamalis, MD

Toxic Anterior Segment Syndrome

Toxic anterior segment syndrome (TASS) is an acute, sterile postoperative anterior segment inflammation that can occur following cataract surgery.[1,2] It is not uncommon for TASS to occur in clusters with several patients affected on the same surgical day.

One of the hallmarks of TASS is the fact that patients present with symptoms within 12 to 48 hours after surgery. It is very important to try and distinguish TASS from possible infectious endophthalmitis. This early onset is a helpful finding because symptoms in infectious endophthalmitis usually develop on average 4 days to 7 days postoperatively. In addition, while some patients may report pain, TASS patients are usually pain free, which is in contrast to infectious endophthalmitis in which up to 75% of the patients complain of pain. The most common clinical findings noted with TASS are marked anterior segment reaction with increased cell and flare, hypopyon formation, and the possibility of fibrin on the surface of the IOL within the pupillary space (Figure 40-1). In addition, widespread "limbus-to-limbus" corneal edema may be seen (Figure 40-2). Other findings may include damage to the iris, which may result in a dilated or irregular pupil, and damage to the trabecular meshwork, which can cause a delayed-onset glaucoma that is oftentimes difficult to treat (Figure 40-3).

Figure 40-1. Anterior segment inflammation with hypopyon formation. (Reprinted from *J Cataract Refract Surg*, 32, Mamalis N, Edelhauser HF, Dawson DG, et al, Toxic anterior segment syndrome (Review/Update), 324-333, Copyright © 2006, with permission of ASCRS and ESCRS.)

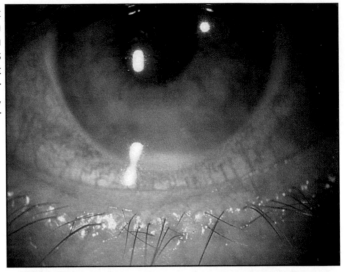

Figure 40-2. Diffuse "limbus-to-limbus" corneal edema. (Reprinted from *J Cataract Refract Surg*, 32, Mamalis N, Edelhauser HF, Dawson DG, et al, Toxic anterior segment syndrome (Review/Update), 324-333, Copyright © 2006, with permission of ASCRS and ESCRS.)

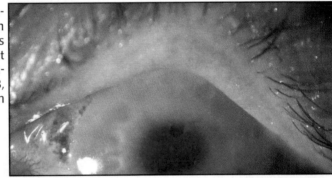

Figure 40-3. Dilated, atrophic iris with irregular pupil. (Reprinted from *J Cataract Refract Surg*, 32, Mamalis N, Edelhauser HF, Dawson DG, et al, Toxic anterior segment syndrome (Review/Update), 324-333, Copyright © 2006, with permission of ASCRS and ESCRS.)

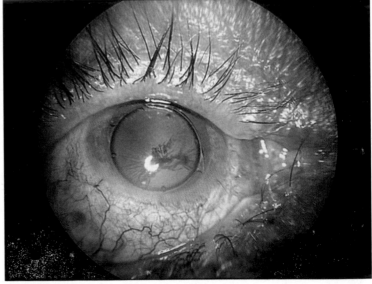

The potential etiologic factors involved in TASS are extremely broad.[3] Problems with any of the solutions or medications that enter the eye during surgery can cause TASS. This includes balanced saline solution (BSS) or any additives placed in the BSS. One of the most common medications added to BSS is epinephrine. It is critical that the epinephrine be free of preservatives (including bisulfites). It is important that intracameral anesthetics such as lidocaine be preservative free and injected in the proper dose. Intracameral antibiotics used any time during the case need to be prepared in the proper doses to ensure that there is no chance of causing toxicity. Lastly, there have been cases of TASS secondary to ophthalmic ointment in the anterior segment of the eye following a clear corneal incision with tight patching, which may cause the wound to gape, allowing access of ointment into the eye.

Another important etiologic factor is the sterilization and preparation of instruments and tubing. Enzyme and detergent residues left on the instruments, especially inside of cannulas or handpieces, can cause toxicity. In addition, endotoxin residues may build up in ultrasound baths or water baths. Because they are heat stable and survive autoclave sterilization, endotoxins remain on instruments and can cause intraocular inflammation if they are injected into the anterior segment of the eye.

It is critically important to ensure that all phacoemulsification and irrigation and aspiration (I/A) handpieces, tips, and cannulas are thoroughly flushed at the conclusion of each case to make sure that there is no residual ophthalmic viscosurgical device (OVD) or cortex left within the lumens.

If a patient is suspected of having TASS, it is important to rule out an infectious etiology. The patient must undergo careful anterior segment evaluation, including slit lamp and gonioscopy. It is essential to assess the severity of the insult to the patient's anterior segment early in the course of his or her condition. The intraocular pressure should be monitored carefully because patients may initially have a low pressure that rapidly climbs secondary to damage to the trabecular meshwork.

The mainstay of treatment for TASS is intense topical corticosteroids. This can include drops of prednisolone acetate 1% on an hourly basis initially. The patient should be followed very carefully during the first several days to ensure that the inflammation is improving during this period of time.

The clinical outcome is often dependent on the severity of the initial insult. Patients with a mild toxin exposure will often show rapid clearing of the inflammation in the anterior segment with little or no residual corneal or iris damage. However, patients with a more severe insult may have persistent corneal edema that may require a cornea transplant. Significant, persistent anterior segment inflammation may lead to problems with secondary glaucoma, pupillary and iris abnormalities, and cystoid macular edema.

Once an outbreak of TASS has been identified, it is critically important for the surgeon and all surgical center or hospital staff members to carefully review all protocols used in the cleaning and sterilization of instruments. It is important that the surgical staff is aware of the potential etiological factors involved with TASS and that all steps are taken to ensure that cannulas, handpieces, and other instruments are thoroughly rinsed with sterile, deionized water at the conclusion of each case. The use of detergents and enzymes within ultrasound baths should be carefully evaluated to ensure that any residue is carefully rinsed from all the instruments and that the water baths are being regularly cleaned and sterilized to ensure that there is no possibility for endotoxin contamination.

Finally, a complete analysis of all medicines and fluids used during the surgery should be undertaken.

It is imperative for surgeons to be aware of the existence of TASS and the steps necessary to treat it and to prevent future occurrences.

References

1. Monson MC, Mamalis N, Olson RJ. Toxic anterior segment inflammation following cataract surgery. *J Cataract Refract Surg.* 1992;18:184-189.
2. Mamalis N. Toxic anterior segment syndrome (Editorial). *J Cataract Refract Surg.* 2006;32:181-182.
3. Mamalis N, Edelhauser HF, Dawson DG, et al. Toxic anterior segment syndrome (Review/Update). *J Cataract Refract Surg.* 2006;32:324-333.

HOW SHOULD I MANAGE PROLONGED OR RECURRENT IRITIS FOLLOWING UNCOMPLICATED SURGERY?

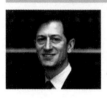

Michael B. Raizman, MD

Patients with unusual amounts of inflammation after cataract surgery require special attention.[1] Two questions should come to mind immediately. 1) Did this patient have iritis any time in the past prior to cataract surgery? 2) Was there an intraoperative complication that could lead to excessive inflammation? The surgeon should always keep in mind the possibility of infectious endophthalmitis.

Patients with preoperative chronic or recurrent iritis are susceptible to unusual amounts of inflammation after routine cataract surgery (Figure 41-1). These patients may require prolonged topical corticosteroid drops after surgery, well beyond the typical 2 weeks to 4 weeks of therapy. More intense inflammation warrants the addition of oral prednisone at an initial dose of approximately 60 mg daily or a 40-mg injection of intraorbital triamcinolone. If patients have a history of uveitis, I wait for the eyes to be quiet for 3 months before performing elective cataract extraction. I usually prescribe prednisone 60 mg daily for 3 days before surgery and for about 1 week or 2 weeks after surgery.

Complicated surgery can lead to increased inflammation. Loss of vitreous, iris prolapse, intraoperative hemorrhage, iris stretching, iris damage, or corneal burns can all lead to unusual amounts of inflammation. Retention of lens fragments may be hard to diagnose. Gonioscopy, B-scan ultrasonography, and anterior segment ultrasound biomicroscopy or optical coherence tomography should be considered to look for retained material. Retained lens fragments in the anterior segment should almost always be removed surgically. These fragments may migrate and damage the corneal endothelium, leading to irreversible corneal edema. Uveitis and glaucoma from retained lens material are also concerns. If the lens material is in the anterior chamber, installation of pilocarpine

Figure 41-1. Causes of postoperative inflammation.

Causes of Excess Postoperative Inflammation

- Preoperative uveitis
- Intraoperative trauma
- Retained lens material
- Endophthalmitis
- IOL irritation of iris or ciliary body

should prevent migration to the posterior chamber and surgical removal should be performed soon. Pieces of lens in the posterior chamber can be more difficult to remove. If the pupil does not dilate widely, then iris hooks may be employed. On the phaco machine, high flow settings with a high bottle height can create turbulence in the eye and encourage pieces of lens to dislodge. Sweeping under the iris with a spatula may be helpful. Intravitreal lens fragments usually need removal but may be observed without surgery if the intraocular pressure is fine and there is no inflammation.

Intraocular lenses may stimulate uveitis if they are not ideally positioned. Mobile lenses are notorious for causing uveitis and cystoid macular edema. A haptic rubbing on the iris or ciliary body can cause inflammation. Anterior chamber lenses should be inspected for iris tuck or migration of a haptic through a peripheral iridectomy.

Excessive postoperative inflammation without prior iritis and without intraoperative complications can occur without warning. Treatment with topical corticosteroids should significantly reduce or eliminate anterior chamber cells. Lack of response to topical therapy or the presence of significant vitreous inflammation should prompt the search for infection. Hypopyon at any time after cataract surgery should suggest infectious endophthalmitis. The capsular bag should be inspected closely for signs of abscess or plaques, but even a clear capsule may harbor bacteria. The presence of vitreal inflammation is always of concern. Any heightened suspicion should lead to a pars plana vitreous tap for culture and simultaneous injection of intravitreal antibiotics. This can be accomplished safely in the office. Broad-spectrum coverage can be achieved with intravitreal vancomycin and ceftazidime. In some cases, the posterior capsule must be opened to allow access of antibiotic to the capsule bag, where the organism is harbored. YAG capsulotomy or pars plana vitrectomy with capsulectomy may be of value prior to antibiotic treatment.

Inflammation may begin many months after cataract surgery in cases of low-grade endophthalmitis. *Propionibacterium acnes* is notorious for this, but it may also arise from staphylococcal, fungal, and other microbial infections.

Cystoid macular edema after routine cataract surgery should be treated with topical prednisolone acetate 4 times a day and a topical nonsteroidal drop at full dose for 4 weeks or longer. The combination of topical corticosteroids and nonsteroidal drops may reduce the incidence of cystoid macular edema after cataract surgery.[2,3] If there is an inadequate resolution, triamcinolone 40 mg may be injected into the orbit. Intravitreal corticosteroids can also be effective. Surgical management of cystoid macular edema is necessary for cases of vitreous traction or poorly positioned intraocular lenses. Cystoid macular edema related to uveitis may not respond as well to topical therapy, and oral corticosteroids or injections may be required.

References

1. Raizman MB. Prolonged Intraocular inflammation. In: Steinert RF, ed. *Cataract Surgery.* 2nd ed. Philadelphia: WB Saunders Co; 2004:601-640.
2. McColgin AZ, Raizman MB. Efficacy of topical Voltaren in reducing the incidence of postoperative cystoid macular edema. *Invest Ophthalmol Vis Sci.* 1999;40:S289.
3. Wittpenn J, et al. Cystoid macular edema after cataract surgery. Paper presented at the American Academy of Ophthalmology Annual Meeting; November 11-14, 2006; New Orleans, La.

FOR HOW LONG CAN I SAFELY OBSERVE A PIECE OF DESCENDED LENS MATERIAL?

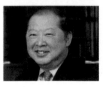

Stanley Chang, MD

Posteriorly dislocated lens fragments are among the more frequently encountered posterior complications during phacoemulsification (Figure 42-1), occurring with a frequency of 0.2% to 0.8% of cases, depending on the experience of the surgeon.[1,2] When this event occurs, it is important to carefully manage the consequences of capsular dehiscence and possible vitreous loss to reduce the potential for retinal complications such as retinal detachment or cystoid macular edema. When posterior capsular rupture or dehiscence is noted and lens fragments migrate into the vitreous, it is helpful to have an adequately dilated pupil, and intracameral epinephrine may be helpful in allowing better visualization. One must decide whether a vitrectomy to remove lens fragments by a vitreoretinal surgeon is feasible at that time. Immediate management objectives include the clearing of any vitreous strands in the anterior chamber and cataract wound, the removal of remaining cortical lens fragments in the capsular bag, and placement of an intraocular lens (IOL).

The extent of any capsular tears should be determined. The use of a fiberoptic endoprobe may illuminate the capsular structures from the side, providing better assessment. In particular, if the posterior capsular tear is small, it might be possible to still remove cortical lens fragments and place the IOL into the capsular bag. If the posterior capsular tear is too large and extends to the equator, the integrity of the anterior capsulorrhexis should be determined and a decision made regarding whether the placement of the IOL into the ciliary sulcus will remain stable. If the capsular bag is significantly separated from zonular attachments and a posterior chamber lens or capsular tension ring cannot be placed, then placement of an anterior chamber lens might be considered. An

Figure 42-1. Posteriorly dislocated lens fragments are one of the more frequently encountered posterior complications during phacoemulsification.

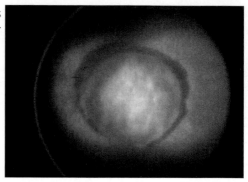

alternative approach would be to suture a posterior chamber IOL to the iris or into the ciliary sulcus. Before placement of the IOL, cortical vitreous in the anterior chamber, the wound, and cortical lens fragments in the capsule should be removed. The IOL may also be placed or sutured after the removal of the dislocated lens fragments with vitrectomy. If the lens nucleus is extremely hard and brunescent, it may be preferable to delay placement of the IOL until after the lens nucleus is removed.

Vitreous in the anterior chamber should be removed with a vitreous cutter. The goal is to clear vitreous strands from the capsular tissues and from the anterior chamber and cataract incision. An anterior infusion sleeve or separate butterfly infusion can be used during the vitrectomy. A standard vitreous cutter at high cutting rates (>1000 cuts/min) should be used at relatively low suction (150 mm Hg for 20-gauge cutters, 400 mm Hg to 500 mm Hg for 25-gauge cutters). A small amount of triamcinolone acetonide (1 mg/mL) might be injected intracamerally to highlight strands of vitreous. The cutter is placed through the limbal cataract incision or can be placed through a pars plana sclerotomy placed 3 mm posterior to the limbus. The anterior vitrectomy can extend posteriorly as far as the cutting port can be visualized. The cutter tip should not proceed posteriorly beyond visualization with the goal of aspirating lens fragments. Directing the irrigation stream posteriorly to force fragments anteriorly during vitrectomy may also be hazardous. Giant retinal tear or dialysis has been associated with overly aggressive anterior vitrectomy and with using the phacoemulsification probe when there is limited visualization.[3]

If fragments of the lens nucleus dislocate posteriorly during cataract surgery, it may be possible to engage a retinal surgeon to perform vitrectomy at the same operation. The anterior segment should be cleared of vitreous and lens debris, and the cornea should be clear enough to allow posterior visualization. The cataract incision should be sutured at least temporarily to allow the infusion to pressurize the globe and avoid a leak or uveal incarceration. A standard vitrectomy with pars plana fragmentation can then be done. If the cornea is not clear, then a delay in surgery is desirable. Not all retained lens fragments require vitrectomy. A few cortical lens fragments may be followed. Indications for vitrectomy to remove posteriorly dislocated lens fragments include excessive inflammation, uncontrolled glaucoma, and rhegmatogenous retinal detachment. Inflammation can be quite severe but a hypopyon is rare from phacolysis. If a hypopyon is present, endophthalmitis should be the primary diagnosis and ruled out. It is possible to wait until inflammation or glaucoma develops postoperatively, but when these develop, vitrectomy should be done promptly. This is important because the associated glaucoma may be difficult to control medically with resultant optic disc damage. Personally, I prefer to operate as soon as possible, usually within the first 1 week to 2 weeks following the phacoemulsification, depending on the clarity of the cornea. The vitrectomy is usually done bimanually with a fiberoptic endoilluminator and the vitrectomy or fragmatome probe. During surgery, the lens fragments can be aspirated and held by the suction of the fragmatome, using the light probe to crush, stabilize, or support the fragments at the ultrasound tip. A useful adjunct is perfluorocarbon liquid, which can be used to provide a protective layer on the retina surface while floating lens fragments anteriorly.

The visual outcomes of vitrectomy for retained lens fragments are generally favorable with 56% to 68% of patients achieving better than 20/40 visual acuity.[4,5] In general, it is believed that the timing of vitrectomy does not seem to influence the final visual outcome. However, in my own experience, eyes with glaucoma or severe inflammation in which surgery is delayed seem to have a longer recovery and are less likely to do well. The most serious complication of dislocated lens fragments is the relatively high rate of retinal detachment, reaching approximately 10% in most published series.[4,6] Thus, it is advisable to perform a careful dilated retinal examination during or shortly after vitrectomy surgery to rule out any retinal tears or dialysis. The visual outcomes are significantly worse if retinal detachments occur. The rate of proliferative vitreoretinopathy is also increased, perhaps because of inflammation caused by the phacolytic process. Other complications that influence the visual outcome are cystoid macular edema, corneal endothelial failure (bullous keratopathy), endophthalmitis, or optic disc pallor (most likely resulting from elevated intraocular pressure).

It is not unusual for the patient to be angry when this complication occurs. It is helpful to explain the situation to the patient and to promptly refer the patient to a retinal specialist. The cataract surgeon should continue to participate in the subsequent management of the patient. Careful attention and a good visual outcome will reduce the likelihood of needing the risk management team later.

References

1. Aasuri MK, Kompella VB, Majji AB. Risk factors for and management of dropped nucleus during phacoemulsification. *J Cataract Refract Surg.* 2001;27:1428-1432.
2. Schwartz SG, Holz ER, Mieler WF, Kuhl DP. Retained lens fragments in resident-performed cataract extractions. *CLAO.* 2002;28:44-47.
3. Aaberg TM Jr, Rubsamen PE, Flynn HW Jr, Chang S, Mieler WF, Smiddy WE. Giant retinal tear as a complication of attempted removal of intravitreal lens fragments during cataract surgery. *Am J Ophthalmol.* 1997;124:222-226.
4. Borne MJ, Tasman W, Regillo C, Malecha M, Sarin L. Outcomes of vitrectomy for retained lens fragments. *Ophthalmology.* 1996;103:971-976.
5. Scott IU, Flynn HW Jr, Smiddy WE, et al. Clinical features and outcomes of pars plana vitrectomy in patients with retained lens fragments. *Ophthalmology.* 2003;110:1567-1572.
6. Salam GA, Greene JM, Deramo VA, Tibrewala RK, Ferrone PJ, Fastenberg DM. Retinal tears and retinal detachment as factors affecting visual outcome after cataract extraction complicated by posteriorly dislocated lens material. *Retina.* 2005;25:570-575.

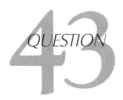

How Should I Manage a Postoperative Refractive Surprise?

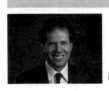

Mark Packer, MD

Most cataract patients and all refractive lens exchange patients expect to achieve spectacle independence for driving and recreation after surgery; those who have opted for presbyopia-correcting intraocular lenses (IOLs) expect to be able to use the computer and read the newspaper without glasses as well. The possibility that an enhancement procedure may be necessary to achieve these goals should be explained to all patients as part of the informed consent process prior to surgery. In addition, they should be provided with information on expected outcomes based on data from relevant Food and Drug Administration (FDA)-monitored clinical studies. For example, 75.7% of subjects bilaterally implanted with the single piece ReStor IOL (SA60D3, Alcon Surgical, Fort Worth, Tex) reported that they never wore glasses (it was 81.0% for the 3-piece MA60D3).[1] Setting realistic expectations is important not only because it lays the foundation for possible postoperative enhancement surgery but also because patients deserve to know the potential risks of surgery.

The most common causes of postoperative refractive surprise include 1) limitations of the precision and accuracy of biometric measurements, 2) the inherent uncertainty of IOL power calculation formulas due to the unpredictability of the final effective lens position, 3) imprecise determination of the corneal power due to previous keratorefractive surgery, and 4) variables such as capsular bag diameter for which no practical and precise measurement technique exists. Several technological solutions are available to reduce the chance of error in biometry and IOL power calculation. Because of its ease of use, superior precision, and repeatability, I prefer partial coherence interferometry (IOLMaster) to measure the axial length. The IOLMaster also provides keratometry, anterior chamber depth, and corneal white-to-white measurements. Immersion A-scan has a continued role, however, for dense cataracts and confirmatory measurements.[2] For enhanced accuracy of corneal power measurements, corneal topography provides simulated keratometry and Effective Refractive Power (Holladay Diagnostic Summary, EyeSys Corneal Analysis System, Tracey Technologies, Houston, Tex). The Holladay IOL Consultant (Jack Holladay, Houston, Tex) provides the benefits of the Holladay II formula as well as regression analysis for personalization of lens constants.

Even with the best available measurements and formulas, refractive surprises can still occur. Management will depend on the patient's expectations. If the error is small and the patient accepts spectacle correction, then the case is closed. There are occasionally situations in which a trial of spectacle or contact lens correction is indicated. I recently had a case of refractive lens exchange with the Crystalens accommodative IOL (AT-45, eyeonics, Inc, Aliso Viejo, Calif) for the correction of high myopia and presbyopia. In keeping with the guidelines of the FDA-approved investigational protocol, the targeted refraction was −0.50 D in the first operated eye (OD) and plano in the second eye (OS). The postoperative refraction in fact remained stable at −0.75 D (20/30, J1 uncorrected visual acuity [UCVA] and 20/15, J2 best-corrected visual acuity [BCVA]) OD and plano (20/20, J2 UCVA) OS. However, the patient was unhappy with his uncorrected distance vision of 20/30 in the right eye. I was concerned that correcting the mild residual myopia in the right eye might deleteriously affect his near vision, so I suggested a monocular contact lens trial. He wore a −0.75-D contact on the right eye for a couple of months and was able to read just fine without additional correction. This result encouraged me to proceed with sulcus piggyback IOL implantation (−1.5 D CLRFLXB, Advanced Medical Optics, Santa Ana, Calif). In the final result, his uncorrected vision in the right eye improved to 20/20 and J1.

As this example illustrates, implantation of a piggyback IOL represents a potential solution for residual spherical refractive error. I will not implant a piggyback IOL until I am certain that the postoperative refractive error is stable. Wait at least 6 weeks after the initial procedure and then obtain 2 refractions at least 2 weeks apart.

Piggyback implantation has advantages of safety and predictability over IOL exchange. It is possible to reopen a fibrotic capsule and explant an IOL even years after surgery[3]; however, implanting a piggyback IOL in the sulcus does not require reopening the capsular bag or cutting and explanting the primary IOL, procedures that put both the capsule and the corneal endothelium at risk. Additionally, exchanging an IOL means implanting a new IOL in the partially fibrosed capsular bag or anterior to the bag in the sulcus; neither location will provide as predictable a postoperative refractive result as a simple piggyback implantation.

Several authors have published simple formulas for calculating the power of a piggyback IOL.[4] For example, Habot-Wilner[5] follows the 1-1 formula described by Holladay for myopic refractive error (power of IOL = desired spherical equivalent change) and chooses the method described by Gills for hyperopic refractive error (power of IOL = [1.4 × desired spherical equivalent change] + 1 D). However, the Holladay IOL Consultant software offers an excellent method for quickly obtaining the desired power (Figure 43-1). In a recent series of 10 piggyback IOL implantations for residual hyperopic error following refractive lens exchange with the Crystalens, Howard Fine, Richard Hoffman, and I achieved excellent predictability using the Holladay R formula (Figure 43-2).

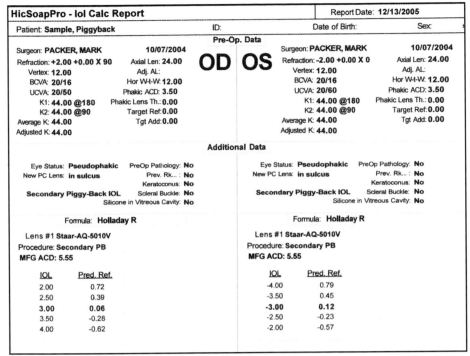

Figure 43-1. Sample output from the Holladay IOL Consultant for piggyback IOL calculation showing a hyperopic refractive error in the right eye and a myopic refractive error in the left eye. Calculations are reported for the STAAR AQ5010V IOL.

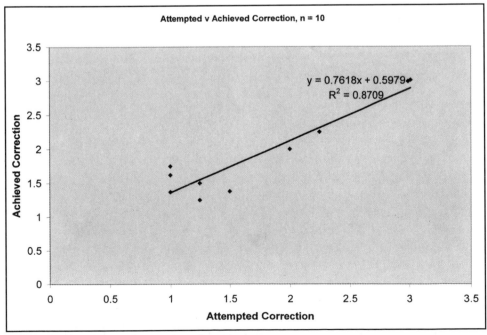

Figure 43-2. Scatter plot of attempted versus achieved correction for piggyback IOL implantation. The Pearson correlation coefficient of 0.8709 demonstrates very high predictability.

Figure 43-3. Shematic diagram of the STAAR AQ5010V IOL.

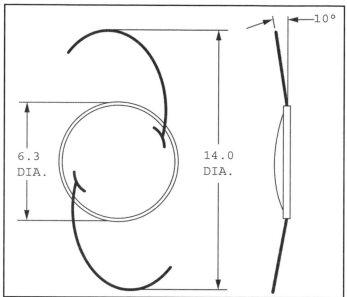

The choice of IOLs for piggyback implantation is limited by the availability of low positive and negative powers in lenses of appropriate design and adequate overall diameter. A sharp or square anterior optic edge and a flat haptic angulation pose increased risk for iris chafing and depigmentation. The round edge, silicone AQ5010V (STAAR Surgical, Monrovia, Calif) is available in whole diopter steps from –4 to +4 (Figure 43-3). It is designed with a 6.3-mm optic, 14.0-mm overall diameter, and a very slim profile that fits well in the sulcus. The silicone CLRFLXB has a rounded anterior edge design ("Opti Edge") and is available from –10 D to +30 D in 0.5-D steps. It has a 6.0-mm optic and 13.0-mm overall diameter. The availability of the CLRFLXB in 0.5-D increments increases the range of choices and the likelihood of achieving the targeted postoperative refraction. The surgical implantation technique for either IOL is straightforward; the piggyback lens optic and both haptics should be placed anterior to the capsule in the sulcus to avoid the chance of interlenticular opacification.[6]

While piggyback IOL implantation represents an elegant solution to the correction of residual spherical refractive errors, it does not address astigmatic correction. Neither toric IOL currently available in the United States is suitable for sulcus placement (STAAR Toric, STAAR, Monrovia, Calif; AcrySof Toric, Alcon, Fort Worth, Tex). For the patient with a significant astigmatic component, lamellar keratorefractive surgical enhancement represents a better solution. I generally prefer laser in situ keratomileusis (LASIK) because of the rapidity of visual rehabilitation (unless contraindicated by corneal dystrophy, pachymetry, suspicious topography, collagen vascular disease, or extreme dry eye syndrome). For patients with a multifocal IOL, great care should be taken in considering wavefront excimer ablation; the wavefront refraction should closely match the manifest refraction if the aberration profile is accurate.[7] In all other respects, the application of LASIK in pseudophakia follows familiar general principles. It provides exceedingly accurate and rapid correction of the small residual refractive errors generally encountered in the postoperative population.

In this era of refractive cataract surgery, it is critical for surgeons to adopt a successful enhancement strategy for the correction of residual refractive errors. Piggyback IOLs and LASIK play important complementary roles in the pursuit of spectacle independence for our patients.

References

1. Summary of safety and effectiveness data. Available at: http://www.fda.gov/cdrh/pdf4/p040020b.pdf. Accessed July 3, 2006.
2. Packer M, Fine IH, Hoffman RS, Coffman PG, Brown LK. Immersion A-scan compared to partial coherence interferometry: outcomes analysis. *J Cataract Refract Surg.* 2002;28:239-242.
3. Fine IH, Hoffman RS. Late reopening of fibrosed capsular bags to reposition decentered intraocular lenses. *J Cataract Refract Surg.* 1997;23(7):990-994.
4. Shepard D. Piggyback intraocular lenses. *Ann Ophthalmol.* 1998;30(4):203-206.
5. Habot-Wilner Z, Sachs D, Cahane M, et al. Refractive results with secondary piggyback implantation to correct pseudophakic refractive errors. *J Cataract Refract Surg.* 2005;31(11):2101-2103.
6. Jackson D. Interlenticular opacification associated with asymmetric haptic fixation of the anterior intraocular lens. *Am J Ophthalmol.* 2003;135(1):106-108.
7. Hardten D. Achieving Success with Refractive IOLs: Clinical Results and Practical Pearls [Course 20-303]. Presented at: Symposium on Cataract, IOL and Refractive Surgery, American Society of Cataract and Refractive Surgery; March 17 to 22, 2006; San Francisco, Calif.

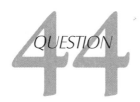

What Causes My Patients to Complain About Temporal Shadows or Reflections, and How Should I Manage Persistent Symptoms?

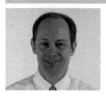

Kevin M. Miller, MD

You perform a perfect cataract operation, the cornea is crystal clear the day after surgery, the patient sees 20/20 or better without glasses, and you hear the nagging word "But!" The patient cups his or her hand on the temporal side of the eye and asks, "Will this go away?" He or she describes a crescent or shadow that is seen as a black arcuate line or band in the temporal field of vision and/or a shimmering or reflection of light.

In retrospect, these visual phenomena were noticed long ago with 5 x 6 mm oval poly-methylmethacrylate (PMMA) intraocular lenses (IOLs), but they became a worldwide nuisance with the introduction of the Alcon 3-piece AcrySof IOL (Fort Worth, Tex). This is the first IOL to have a square edge design containing sharp anterior and posterior bends (Figure 44-1). The edge was designed that way for manufacturing convenience, but it was found in clinical practice to produce the beneficial effect of lowering or slowing the rate of posterior capsule opacification. The square edge quickly became the gold standard for lens edge design by all manufacturers despite the reports of adverse visual phenomena that were popping up all around. The AcrySof lens was manufactured in acrylic, but its edge design was quickly copied into IOLs made of silicone, collamer, and other materials. The visual phenomena that all of these lenses produce are related primarily to edge architecture. However, material is also important, with symptoms simply being more apparent when high index of refraction acrylic is used.

There are many lens-related visual disturbances. The American Academy of Ophthalmology's Basic and Clinical Science Course text on Clinical Optics, for which I am the recent past writing committee chairman, provides a brief review of this subject.[1]

Figure 44-1. This scanning electron microscope image shows the original 3-piece Alcon AcrySof IOL that produced unwanted visual disturbances because of its square edge design. (Reprinted from *J Cataract Refract Surg, 26,* Tester R, Pace NL, Samore M, Olson RJ, Dysphotopsia in phakic and pseudophakic patients: incidence and relation to intraocular lens type, 810-816, © 2000, with permission from ASCRS & ESCRS.)

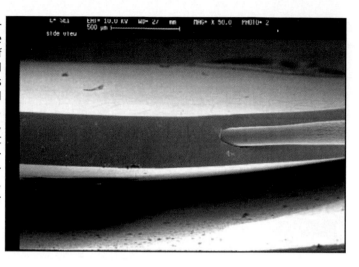

I outlined my thoughts on this topic for the *Journal of Cataract and Refractive Surgery* as well.[2] Our current discussion will be limited to aberrations induced by lens edges only. I prefer to name the phenomenon described by the typical patient edge scotoma and edge reflection. Randall Olson and colleagues at the University of Utah coined the term *dysphotopsia* to describe the symptoms.[3] I do not like this word for a couple of reasons. By its nature, any photopsia is a "dys" in that it is unpleasant and unwanted; the prefix is redundant. Additionally, normal photopsias arise in the absence of light. The phenomena that patients with square edge lenses experience occur only in the presence of light, not in its absence. Despite my objections, the term *dysphotopsia* has been repeated so many times in the literature that we will probably have to live with it for now.

It is hard to define the incidence of lens edge-related visual phenomena. In visually attentive young healthy patients whose pupils dilate well, it may be as high as 15% to 20%. In older patients with smaller pupils, the incidence is lower. It is more common in patients implanted with acrylic as opposed to silicone and collamer IOLs and more common when the optic diameter of a lens is small. Lenses with 5.0-mm and 5.5-mm optics are much more likely to produce visual symptoms than lenses with 6-mm optics. I saw this early on in my 3-piece AcrySof experience.

What produces these annoying visual phenomena? They are easy to understand once you refer to Figure 44-2. First, the symptoms are usually apparent only on the temporal side of vision because only this side allows light to enter the eye obliquely enough to strike the edge of the IOL. The forehead or brow, nose, and cheek block the oblique entry of light in other quadrants. Light from the mid to far periphery on the temporal side of the visual field enters the pupil and strikes the edge of the lens. The light is more likely to gain access to the edge of the IOL if the pupil is large or the diameter of the optic is small. The flat edge of the IOL acts like a plano mirror. Some of the light reflects off the edge and is scattered toward the temporal side of the eye. This light is unavailable to pass through the edge, so it creates an arcuate shadow on the nasal retina. The brain interprets this shadow as a dark crescent or scotoma in the temporal visual field. The light that reflects to the opposite side of the eye is seen as a shimmer or light flash. The shadow is the temporal scotoma or negative dysphotopsia. The reflected light is the edge reflection or positive dysphotopsia.

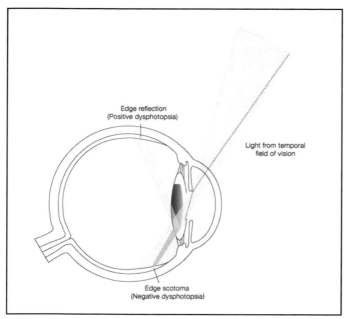

Edge reflection
(Positive dysphotopsia)

Light from temporal
field of vision

Edge scotoma
(Negative dysphotopsia)

Figure 44-2. This diagram explains the origin of edge scotoma and edge reflection produced by square edge IOLs. (Reprinted from *J Cataract Refract Surg, 31,* Miller KM, Consultation section reply, 1488-1489, © 2005, with permission from ASCRS & ESCRS.)

The only certain way to avoid lens edge aberrations is to implant IOLs with low refractive indices, large diameter optics, and round edges. Older style silicone IOLs fit this description, but they have a high incidence of posterior capsule opacification and fibrosis. Since square edge lens aberrations are worse when lenses decenter, IOLs should be placed in the capsular bag whenever possible and zonular laxity should be managed, giving consideration to implantation of a capsular tension ring if necessary. If for any reason an IOL must be implanted in the ciliary sulcus, IOLs with square edges should be avoided. My lens of choice for the ciliary sulcus is the STAAR Surgical model AQ2010V (Monrovia, Calif). This is a 3-piece foldable silicone IOL with a round edge.

What should you do if a patient complains postoperatively? First, I assure my patients that this is a common problem experienced by 15% to 20% of patients. I tell them that it will likely go away in several weeks to months if they wait it out. As the peripheral capsule fibroses around the edge of the lens, the edge reflection and temporal scotoma problems will diminish. I polish the anterior capsules of my cataract patients using Shepherd anterior capsule polishers (Momentum Medical Inc, Tampa, Fla), so the resolution of their symptoms is delayed, but I do this because it helps keep their anterior capsule clear and reduces the incidence of IOL decentration. If adequate time has elapsed and a patient continues to complain, a trial of Alphagan P (Allergan, Inc, Irvine, Calif) or dilute pilocarpine is reasonable. I do not think pharmacologic measures are a good long-term solution, however. The ultimate solution for lens edge aberrations is IOL exchange, substituting a round edge design for the square edge lens. A 3-piece silicone or STAAR Surgical collamer plate-haptic IOL can be implanted. If a plate-haptic lens is chosen, the plate should be oriented in the 180-degree meridian so that the square edge lies out in the periphery of the capsular bag. We have successfully performed many IOL exchanges to resolve patients' symptoms.[4] There are anecdotal oral reports of plano piggyback silicone IOL implantation in the sulcus, but I can think of no optical reason why this should work. In fact, pushing the primary lens posteriorly might actually worsen the visual symptoms because the lens edge will become visible to light entering the eye at more acute angles.

If there is any question as to whether an IOL exchange will be necessary to resolve symptoms, every effort should be made to delay or avoid a laser capsulotomy until the lens edge symptoms disappear or at least 6 months has elapsed. If an IOL exchange is necessary, it will be much easier to perform in the absence of a posterior capsulotomy.

Most patients with lens-related visual disturbances simply need to be reassured that their problems will diminish with time. They can be told that IOL exchange will eliminate the symptoms if they do not disappear on their own.

References

1. Clinical Optics. Basic and Clinical Science Course. San Francisco: American Academy of Ophthalmology; 2005:222-224.
2. Miller KM. Consultation section reply. *J Cataract Refract Surg.* 2005;31:1488-1489.
3. Tester R, Pace NL, Samore M, Olson RJ. Dysphotopsia in phakic and pseudophakic patients: incidence and relation to intraocular lens type. *J Cataract Refract Surg.* 2000;26:810-816.
4. Farbowitz MA, Zabriskie NA, Crandall AS, Olson RJ, Miller KM. Visual complaints of patients with AcrySof intraocular lenses. *J Cataract Refract Surg.* 2000;26:1339-1345.

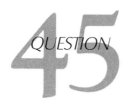
WHAT SHOULD I DO ABOUT THE SECOND EYE IN A PATIENT COMPLAINING ABOUT SEVERE HALOS AFTER THE FIRST MULTIFOCAL?

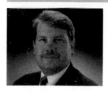

Kevin L. Waltz, OD, MD

The most important question to ask is, "Are the patient's complaints related to problems that will likely resolve with time, will they require an intervention, or are the complaints of a type and severity that the patient will not adapt to them?" If you believe the patient will improve with time, then you support the patient emotionally while he or she continues to improve. If you believe the symptoms are not resolvable, then it is best to perform an intraocular lens (IOL) exchange within 1 month to 2 months after the surgery date.

The timing of an IOL exchange is important. An IOL exchange is an uncommon procedure for most surgeons, but it can be accomplished with consistently good results with proper training and planning. It is easier to exchange an IOL within 1 month of implantation. It is possible to exchange an IOL for many months or years after implantation. The relative risk can be predicted by stability of the zonules and the degree of fibrosis of the capsule to the multifocal IOL. A useful pearl for IOL exchange is to lift the existing IOL out of the capsular bag and into the anterior chamber, then place the second or replacement IOL into the capsular bag underneath the first IOL. Doing so increases the protection of the capsule and effectively increases the safe working dimensions of the anterior chamber as the original IOL is removed. When you exchange a multifocal IOL, it is usually best to replace it with a monofocal IOL and not another multifocal IOL.

Prior to exchanging a multifocal IOL for a monofocal IOL, you should consider proceeding with the second eye surgery. This can sometimes be challenging when the patient is experiencing severe halos in the first eye. When a patient complains of severe halos after an initial multifocal IOL implantation, you can propose using a different multifocal IOL or a wavefront-corrected monofocal IOL in the second eye. The monofocal IOL will reduce the risk of halos in the second eye. The combination of a multifocal IOL in one eye and a monofocal IOL in the other eye will give the patient useful distance and near vision in the multifocal eye with the "cost" of halos and great distance vision without halos in the other eye with the "cost" of poor near vision. The combination, with the benefits of binocular vision, will frequently provide good distance and near vision with significantly less symptomatic halos as compared to having bilateral multifocal IOLs.

The symptoms of severe halos are specific. The halos seen at distance by patients with multifocal IOLs are caused by the near portion of the IOL focusing light in front of the retina. The patient is aware of a ring of light around an object, which can take one of several forms. The ring is a donut of light separated from the object by a clear space. This description is typical of individual points of lights with dark backgrounds, like stars. There can be a "glow" around the object. This is seen when many individual points of light are close together and form a larger object, which is essentially many point sources of light that cluster together, like the moon.

Halos are a form of spherical aberration. If you look on the Zernike pyramid, you will see halos as the pattern representing spherical aberration (SA). We all develop SA as we age. This is one of the main reasons you will have patients come to you in their 40s with uncorrected distance visual acuity of 20/15 or greater with complaints of poor vision. The patient used to have a better visual quality, but they developed SA as they aged. The progressive SA has caused an associated loss of contrast sensitivity and some patients will notice it.

The phenomenon of increasing SA with age is helpful to understand for lens surgery patients. This is one of the reasons a patient who is age 60 is more likely to accept the compromise of multifocal vision than a patient who is 50. The 60-year-old patient has experienced more SA from his or her natural lens prior to lens surgery and adapts more quickly to the halos of a multifocal IOL than a younger patient who has not experienced as much SA.

The patient's tolerance of the halos will always improve over time from neuroadaptation. Neuroadaptation is a poorly understood, but very real adjustment that the patient's mind makes to undesirable images such as halos. The images presented in this chapter are a classic example of the ability of a multifocal patient to mentally erase an unwanted image (Figure 45-1). This patient is drawing the images her mind sees over time. The image quality improves over time. It is very likely this improvement comes from improved mental processing of the image and not a physical change in the image. If the patient has experienced more SA prior to his or her surgery, he or she will adapt to the SA or halos of a multifocal IOL more rapidly.

Greater SA prior to lens surgery is associated with increased age, increasing amounts of hyperopia, prior laser vision correction, and larger pupil size. SA can also be directly measured preoperatively and postoperatively with a wavefront analyzer. It is common for a patient with hyperopia prior to surgery to report that the halos of a multifocal IOL are less bothersome than the halos noted from their natural lens.

Pupil size is a major determinant of halo severity. Smaller pupils are associated with less SA. Making a pupil smaller with medications will usually make the halos less symptomatic. It is always appropriate to try brimonidine to temporarily make the pupil smaller.

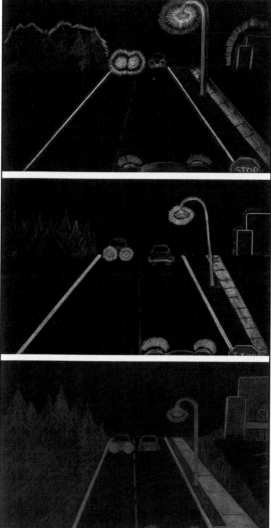

Figure 45-1. These three images demonstrate the gradual neuroadaptation to the halos of a multifocal IOL over time. All images are drawn by an artist patient of Dr. Michael Woodcock. The top image is immediately postoperative and shows relatively dramatic halos. The middle image is several months postoperative and shows the halos are significantly reduced. The bottom image is several years postoperative and shows the halos essentially gone. This is a typical progression of neuroadaptation reported by most patients. (Courtesy of Dr. Michael Woodcock.)

Brimonidine will usually reduce the pupil diameter by about 1 mm with a slightly greater effect in lower illumination. This will lessen the degree of halo symptoms and will give you an idea of how bothersome the halo is to the patient. You will often hear the patient say that brimonidine decreases the halo, but it is too much trouble to use the drop once a day. Diluted pilocarpine of 0.5% or 1% can also be used to decrease the halo. Pilocarpine will reduce the pupil size much more than brimonidine and patients will usually report better vision at distance and near due to the pinhole effect. The pilocarpine pinhole effect may effectively improve symptoms related to residual astigmatism as well. Long-term pilocarpine use after lens surgery may be associated with an elevated risk of retinal detachment in previously myopic eyes.

Residual refractive error after implantation of a multifocal IOL has a significant effect on postoperative symptoms. An eye with residual myopia will have significant halos. An eye that is left hyperopic will have decreased near vision in proportion to the residual hyperopia. Residual astigmatism superimposed over the spherical refractive error will make the halos or blur even worse. It is not possible to achieve the desired refractive end point after lens surgery in every case. Therefore, you can expect that eyes implanted with a multifocal lens will occasionally require laser vision correction (LVC) enhancement to improve uncorrected vision and to decrease symptoms such as halos related to residual myopia.

Conventional LVC is the preferred method for enhancing eyes implanted with a multifocal IOL. Custom LVC with currently available algorithms can create unpredictable problems with currently available multifocal IOLs. LCV is usually done 1 month to 3 months after implantation of a multifocal IOL. Implantation of a multifocal IOL in an eye with previous custom or conventional LVC is not contraindicated.

Bibliography

Agarwal A, ed. *Presbyopia: A Surgical Textbook.* Thorofare, NJ: SLACK Incorporated; 2002.
Belville JK, Smith RJ. *Presbyopia Surgery: Pearls and Pitfalls.* Thorofare, NJ: SLACK Incorporated; 2006.
Tzubota K, Boxer Wachler BS, Azar D, Koch D. *Hyperopia and Presbyopia.* New York: Marcel Dekker; 2003.

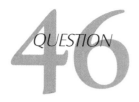
CAN I MIX DIFFERENT MULTIFOCAL INTRAOCULAR LENSES OR MULTIFOCAL WITH MONOFOCAL INTRAOCULAR LENSES?

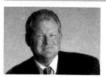

Richard L. Lindstrom, MD

Multifocal intraocular lenses and accommodating intraocular lenses can be paired with a normal crystalline lens in the opposite eye, a monofocal implant in the opposite eye, or a different multifocal or accommodating lens in the opposite eye. Combining complementary intraocular lenses provides a superior outcome to that achieved utilizing the same implant in both eyes.

The concept of using different optical systems that are complementary in each of a patient's eyes is not new. The most common example of this, familiar to all ophthalmologists, is monovision in which 1 eye is set for distance and the other for near. If the difference between the 2 eyes is greater than 1.50 D, I call that monovision and if it is less than 1.5 D, I call it blended vision. In blended vision, some stereopsis and fusion are retained and a relative amblyopia for distance is less likely.

In the case of multifocal and accommodating lenses, there are at least 10 potential options that can be utilized:

1. An accommodating lens can be implanted into 1 eye and a normal crystalline lens in the opposite eye.

2. A multifocal lens can be implanted into 1 eye and a normal crystalline lens in the other eye.

3. Bilateral accommodating intraocular lenses can be utilized with a symmetrical refractive outcome target.

4. Bilateral accommodating intraocular lens can be utilized with a blended vision outcome (eg, targeting −0.25 D in 1 eye and −1.00 D in the alternate eye).

5. Bilateral multifocal implants with the same optical configuration can be implanted in both eyes with a symmetrical refractive outcome target.

6. Bilateral multifocal implants with the same optical configuration can be utilized with a blended vision outcome (eg, targeting plano in 1 eye and −0.50 D in the alternate eye).

7. An accommodating intraocular lens can be implanted in 1 eye and a monofocal implant in the opposite eye.

8. A multifocal intraocular lens can be implanted in 1 eye and the monofocal lens in the opposite eye.

9. An accommodating intraocular lens can be implanted in 1 eye and a multifocal lens in the opposite eye.

10. Complementary multifocal intraocular lenses can be implanted in the alternate eyes (eg, a zonal aspheric intraocular multifocal intraocular lens [ReZoom, Advanced Medical Optics, Santa Ana, Calif] in 1 eye and an apodized diffractive/refractive multifocal intraocular lens in the opposite eye [ReSTOR, Alcon, Fort Worth, Tex]). This has become known as "mixing and matching" presbyopia-correcting intraocular lenses.

In order to best use complementary intraocular lenses, it is important that the ophthalmologist understand the strengths and weaknesses of each intraocular lens.

The standard monofocal intraocular lens is the best economic value. It gives excellent distance, fair intermediate, and poor near vision (eg, 20/20+, J4, J7 at the 3 distances, respectively). The pseudoaccommodative amplitude is approximately 2 D, which means it has about 1 D of pseudoaccommodative amplitude to the minus side. This means that if the patient is targeted for a −1.50 refractive outcome, he or she will be able to read as though he or she had a +2.00 to +2.50 reader. The lens has positive spherical aberration of approximately +0.10 μm, somewhat dependent on optic power and optic design. This type of spherical aberration is best in patients who have negative spherical aberrations in the cornea such as those posthyperopic laser in situ keratomileusis (LASIK), with keratoconus, or with a cornea with naturally occurring negative spherical aberration (10% to 20%).

Second, we have aspheric monofocal intraocular lenses, including those with no spherical aberration (Bausch & Lomb's Advanced Optic, Rochester, NY) and those with negative spherical aberration (Advanced Medical Optics' TECNIS, Santa Ana, Calif and Alcon IQ, Fort Worth, Tex). The intraocular lens with no spherical aberration is most forgiving of decentration and tilt and might be selected in patients where decentration might occur such as in pseudoexfoliation, a capsular tear, or where an ideal capsulorrhexis is not available.

The implants with negative spherical aberration give better quality of vision, especially under mesopic conditions, in the patient with a typical cornea with positive corneal spherical aberration. They also provide superior performance in the patient that has undergone myopic keratorefractive surgery.

The Eyeonics' Crystalens (Aliso Viejo, Calif) is an accommodating intraocular lens that gives excellent distance and intermediate vision. Typically, one can achieve 20/20+ and

J1 at distance and intermediate, respectively. It provides good near acuity with a typical outcome being J3 or better. This lens produces the least night vision symptoms, the least loss of contrast sensitivity, and the least color distortion of all currently available presbyopia-correcting intraocular lenses. It is also pupil-size independent in its optical function and is excellent for blended vision.

The ReZoom, a zonal aspheric multifocal intraocular lens manufactured by AMO, provides good distance acuity, good intermediate acuity, and good near acuity. Typical outcomes are 20/20 distance, J2 intermediate, and J2 at near. There are some night vision symptoms, some loss of contrast sensitivity, and some color distortion with this IOL. The refractive performance of this lens is pupil-size dependent.

The AMO Multifocal TECNIS, an aspheric diffractive multifocal intraocular lens, provides good distance acuity, fair intermediate, and excellent near acuity. Typical outcomes to be expected are 20/20- at distance, J4 at intermediate, and J1 at near. It also has the potential for night vision symptoms, decreased contrast sensitivity, and some color distortion. The decreased contrast sensitivity usually associated with a multifocal implant is reduced by the aspheric nature of the optic. The refractive performance of this lens is not pupil-size dependent.

The Alcon ReSTOR, an apodized diffractive/refractive multifocal intraocular lens, provides good distance acuity, fair intermediate, and excellent near. Distance acuity might be expected to be 20/20-, intermediate J4, and near J1. This lens also potentially generates night vision symptoms, decreased contrast sensitivity, and color distortion. Its refractive performance is also pupil-size dependent because the lens becomes more distance dominant as the pupil dilates.

The author and other members of his practice (Minnesota Eye Consultants, PA) have utilized all of the above combinations of implants with good success. Multifocal intraocular lenses have been used in a mix-and-match approach for approximately 20 years, beginning in 1985. Our experience has been that almost all patients adapt well over time to the use of complementary optics in their alternate eyes.

Neuroadaptation is a concept that is receiving increased attention as ophthalmologists use more and more optical systems that are dissimilar to the natural crystalline lens. It appears that there is both an early stage and late stage neuroadaptation. Approximately 80% of patients seem to adapt easily to complementary optics whereas 20% may struggle for a few months to a year or more. Late neuroadaptation appears to occur at near 100% and the author's personal experience is that there are no patients in his practice with over 2 years follow-up with dissimilar optics who have not adapted well to their optical system.

Recent clinical series of "mixing and matching" some multifocal and accommodating intraocular lenses provide insight into the outcomes that might be obtained. Leonardo Akaishi, MD and Pedro Paulo Fabri, from Sao Paulo, Brazil have performed a comparative series of ReZoom/ReZoom, ReSTOR/ReSTOR, ReZoom/ReSTOR, and TECNIS Diffractive/ReZoom. Their outcomes are summarized in Table 46-1. The best outcomes were obtained with ReZoom/ReSTOR and ReZoom/TECNIS diffractive intraocular lens combinations.

Rick Milne, MD from Columbia, SC has also performed a comparative series looking at patient satisfaction, spectacle independence, and daytime and nighttime halo. His outcomes are summarized in Table 46-2. Again, the ReZoom/ReSTOR outcomes generated higher patient satisfaction than the ReSTOR/ReSTOR outcomes in this series.

Table 46-1

Comparative Series of ReZoom/ReZoom, ReSTOR/ReSTOR, ReZoom/ReSTOR, and TECNIS Diffractive/ReZoom

	ReZoom/ReZoom (N = 100)	ReSTOR/ReSTOR (N = 100)	ReZoom/ReSTOR (N = 88)	ReZoom/Tecnis Diffractive (N = 15)
Bilateral uncorrected distance	20/20	20/25	20/20	20/20
Bilateral uncorrected intermediate	J2.15	J3.85	J2.30	J2.10
Bilateral uncorrected near	J2.30	J1.40	J1.50	J1.10
Average reading speed (words per minute)	125	165	155	185
Spectacle independence	75%	89%	100%	100%
Halos/glare	2+	1+	1+	1-
MTF	0.20	0.12	0.18	0.38

Table 46-2

Comparative Series of Patient Satisfaction, Spectacle Independence, and Daytime and Nighttime Halo

	ReSTOR/ReSTOR (N = 30+)	ReZoom/ReSTOR (N = 30+)
Satisfied/very satisfied	83%	96%
Neutral dissatisfied	0%	4%
Very dissatisfied	17%	0%
Would have procedure again, recommend to family and friends	70%	97%
Complete spectacle independence	65%	94%
Daytime halo	43%	18%
Nighttime halo	86%	71%
Requesting explants	6%	0%

Table 46-3
Comparative Series of ReSTOR/ReSTOR to ReZoom/ReZoom

	ReSTOR/ReSTOR *(N = 55+)*	*ReZoom/ReSTOR* *(N = 39+)*	
Bilateral uncorrected distance	20/25	20/25	(P = NS)
Bilateral uncorrected intermediate	J3.81	J2.39	(P.001)
Bilateral uncorrected near	J1.00	J1.04	(P = NS)
Unhappy with intermediate	32%	0%	

Table 46-4
Comparative Series of Patients With Crystalens/ReSTOR Use in Alternate Eyes

	Crystalens/ReSTOR (N = 32)
Bilateral uncorrected distance	20/25
Bilateral uncorrected intermediate	J1.3
Bilateral uncorrected near	J1.3

Frank A. Bucci, Jr, MD from Wilkes-Barre, Penn has also completed a series comparing ReSTOR/ReSTOR to ReZoom/ReZoom. His outcomes are summarized in Table 46-3. Of note is that his intermediate vision outcomes are significantly better with ReZoom/ReSTOR than with ReSTOR/ReSTOR and that his patient satisfaction is also higher.

Finally, Trevor Woodhams, MD from Atlanta, Ga has a series of patients with Crystalens/ReSTOR use in alternate eyes (Table 46-4). Again, he found excellent distance, intermediate, and near vision with high patient satisfaction.

Conclusion

The human visual system can neuroadapt to dissimilar optics in alternate eyes. Patients should be given at least 1 year to neuroadapt to their new optical system before explant/exchange is considered. Multifocal or accommodating intraocular lenses can be used successfully with a monofocal intraocular lens in the opposite eye. Multifocal or accommodating intraocular lenses can also be used successfully with a natural crystalline lens in the opposite eye. Of great importance is the observation that complementary multifocal and accommodating intraocular lenses may provide superior outcomes for many patients compared to symmetrical implantation of the same intraocular lens in both eyes. This is particularly true for function at intermediate distance. Further clinical study is ongoing, but the current evidence supports the use of complementary presbyopia-correcting intraocular lenses in the alternate eyes of select patients.

Bibliography

Davis EA, Hardten DH, Lindstrom RL. *Presbyopic Lens Surgery: A Clinical Guide to Current Technology.* Thorofare, NJ: SLACK Incorporated; 2007.

Lindstrom RL. Foreword. In: Holladay JT, ed. *Quality of Vision: Essential Optics for the Cataract and Refractive Surgeon.* Thorofare, NJ: SLACK Incorporated; 2006.

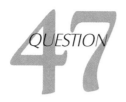
Following a Posterior Capsular Rent, the Sulcus-Fixated Intraocular Lens Has Become Decentered. How Should I Proceed?

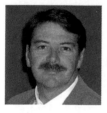

Garry P. Condon, MD

Cause and Prevention

Intraocular lens (IOL) decentration is a common and often puzzling problem occurring days to years after attempted IOL placement in the sulcus because of a posterior capsule tear. In the presence of an intact anterior capsulorrhexis, possible causes for decentration include inadequate IOL length for a large sulcus diameter, a localized zonular defect, haptic damage, or haptic memory loss. With a discontinuous capsulorrhexis, the subluxation of the IOL may often be caused by asymmetric bag/sulcus haptic positions aggravated by late contraction of the residual capsule complex. In either case, associated vitreous prolapse or incarceration can contribute to the IOL malposition and can cause a pupil deformity.

The intraoperative duress of dealing with a posterior capsule rent often clouds our thinking to the degree that we are happy to simply get the IOL in the sulcus. However, we can usually prevent subsequent IOL decentration by prolapsing the optic posteriorly through an intact anterior capsulorrhexis to capture it while leaving the haptics in the sulcus. The importance of this simple maneuver cannot be overemphasized because it also prevents vitreous prolapse and pigment dispersion caused by the optic chafing the iris.

Treatment Options

I recommend intervention for a decentered IOL primarily for intolerable visual symptoms. Indications include reduced visual acuity, glare, edge effect halos, and photophobia as well as complications like uveitis-glaucoma-hyphema syndrome and cystoid macular edema.[1] The options include observation, miotics, or surgery with repositioning, exchange, or explantation of the IOL. Many of these IOLs remain in a mildly decentered but stable location requiring only observation. I have found patient-directed miotic therapy with 1% pilocarpine to be useful for mild decentration that is often only symptomatic at night. In those needing surgical therapy for an out-of-the-bag decentered IOL, I prefer simple repositioning or peripheral iris suture fixation of the haptics. I reserve IOL exchange as a last option.

Preoperative Evaluation

The preoperative evaluation must include a detailed slit-lamp examination attempting to determine the actual position of the IOL in relation to any residual capsule layers. Preoperative gonioscopy may further enhance visualization. However, I often find it impossible to determine the amount of available capsule support and its degree of continuity until I am in the operating room where I am able to retract iris for an optimal view. Predilated and postdilated examinations best reveal iris anatomy and pupil function and the need to perform a pupilloplasty as part of the surgery.

While sometimes difficult, it is important to determine the material and design of the decentered IOL. A large single piece polymethylmethacrylate (PMMA) IOL may be best suited to scleral fixation as opposed to a 3-piece design with flexible haptics, which I prefer suturing to the iris. I attempt to get the original IOL power and routinely include biometry in evaluating all of these cases. Unanticipated IOL exchange is always a possibility.

Instrumentation

For simple repositioning or suture fixation, a small diamond knife enables me to make paracenteses without deforming the globe. While a Sinsky hook, a Kuglen hook, and an iris spatula are all valuable, I find the recently available anterior segment microforceps from Microsurgical Technologies, Inc (Redmond, Wash) dramatically improves my ability to manipulate the IOL, iris, and capsule during surgery (Figure 47-1). Disposable nylon iris retractors are invaluable devices to not only improve visualization while suturing but to support the IOL haptic itself during fixation. I prefer viscoelastic agents, such as Healon (Advanced Medical Optics, Santa Ana, Calif) or Provisc (Alcon, Fort Worth, Tex), that are easy to remove completely through small incisions with simple irrigation. This reduces the risk of postoperative intraocular pressure elevation. The suture material I use for iris fixation is 10-0 polypropylene on a long curved needle, such as the PC-7 (Alcon, Fort Worth, Tex), the CIF-4 (Ethicon, Cornelia, Ga), or the CTC-6 (Ethicon, Cornelia, Ga). I use 9-0 polypropylene for scleral fixation.

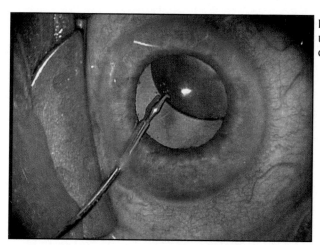

Figure 47-1. A 23-gauge microforcep is used to grasp and manipulate a dislocated IOL.

Surgical Techniques

The first question to consider before surgery is how widely the pupil should be dilated. While mydriasis improves our view of the IOL position and available support, I often want to create temporary pupillary capture of the optic as part of the procedure. For this reason, I prefer topical 1% tropicamide and 2.5% phenylephrine because they still allow for a good response to intracameral acetylcholine to constrict the pupil when needed. Even without preoperative mydriasis, intracameral lidocaine can dilate the pupil adequately early on, while still allowing it to respond to acetylcholine.

The simplest form of decentered sulcus IOL management is manipulation with reorientation of the haptics into meridians where capsule and zonule support appears adequate. I consider this a viable option when there is at least 270 degrees of contiguous support. A combination of Sinsky and Kuglen hooks placed through paracentesis tracts are used within viscoelastic to rotate the optic and haptics. There is always a tendency for the IOL to rotate back to the meridian lacking sulcus support and eventually decenter again. In these seemingly simple cases, I like to place a single peripheral McCannel suture to fixate one haptic to the iris to prevent rotation and secure the desired orientation. This is somewhat analogous to the effect of a steering wheel lock.

The majority of freely mobile out-of-the-bag IOLs are best managed with peripheral iris suture fixation of the haptics using a modified McCannel approach with some form of Siepser sliding knots.[2,3] I begin with mild pharmacologic dilation followed by topical tetracaine and intracameral 1.5% lidocaine mpf for anesthesia. A nonretentive viscoelastic is used to stabilize anterior chamber depth and encase the IOL for support during manipulation. I am careful to not overinflate the chamber to best achieve a planar iris contour. I then bring the optic anterior to the pupil with either hooks or a microforceps and attempt to capture it with the pupil. I will often add the acetylcholine with one hand through the side port while supporting the IOL with the other hand. Capturing the optic by the pupil is the key maneuver and is generally manageable with any 3-piece IOL and reasonable pupil anatomy (Figure 47-2). Following optic capture, the addition of viscoelastic over the iris in the region of the peripheral haptics will easily delineate the actual haptic location and facilitate accurate suture passage. At this point, I select an appropriate limbal

Figure 47-2A. A combination of hooks are used to bring the optic above the iris plane for capture.

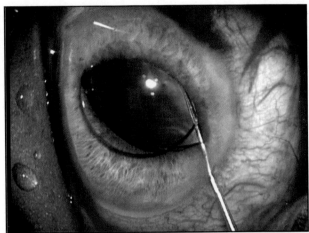

Figure 47-2B. Capture is completed with the addition of acetylcholine to induce miosis.

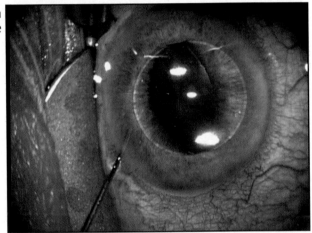

paracentesis site to introduce the suture. I find it works best to create the entry paracentesis for the needle about 1 to 2 clock hours away from the actual peripheral haptic location. The paracentesis should be just inside the limbus and oriented fairly tangential to it. These factors allow good visualization of the needle tip as it is passed through the iris and avoid an overly steep needle angle. Once the needle is passed through the peripheral iris and behind the haptic, simply lifting the needle slightly should create movement of the entire IOL, confirming that I will have the haptic included in the suture bite. I bring the needle tip up through the iris and directly out through any nearby area of clear cornea (Figure 47-3). Although the 2 suture ends can be retrieved through another common paracentesis created over the haptic to complete a knot, I find a Siepser sliding knot technique provides more precise knot tensioning and better security.[4] The second haptic is fixed in this same manner and the optic is prolapsed back into the posterior chamber.

I consider repairing a deformed pupil either prior to attempting optic capture or at the conclusion of the IOL fixation. In cases associated with moderate traumatic mydriasis, I prefer pupilloplasty as an initial step to improve subsequent capture of the IOL optic. Any vitreous prolapse must be managed using proper vitrectomy instrumentation. I use the handpiece without an irrigating sleeve and obtain inflow via an anterior chamber-maintaining cannula.

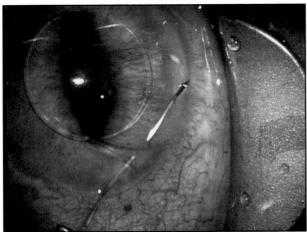

Figure 47-3A. The needle has been passed through the paracentesis, through the iris, behind the haptic, back out through the iris and through an area of distal clear cornea.

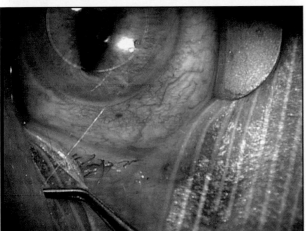

Figure 47-3B. A Siepser sliding knot is preferred in this case to secure the haptics to the peripheral iris.

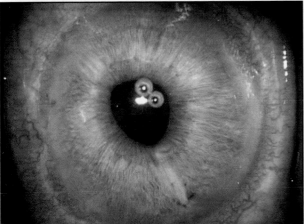

Figure 47-3C. After the haptics are secured, the optic is prolapsed back into the posterior chamber and the sutures are barely visible in the periphery at the 5:00 and 10:00 positions.

Unlike a 3-piece IOL, achieving temporary optic capture of large single piece PMMA IOL is often more challenging because the large diameter and more rigid haptics tend to keep the entire lens trapped posterior to the ciliary body. This can create severe posterior vaulting away from the pupil plane. I usually consider ab externo scleral fixation for these cases. I create a conjunctiva peritomy at the site of a desired fixation point and a midperipheral cornea paracentesis is made 180 degrees away. A hollow 26-gauge needle is placed through the sclera at the desired fixation site within a shallow scleral groove 1.5 mm behind the limbus. The tip of the needle is brought into the pupillary zone. One end of a double-arm 9-0 polypropylene suture on a long needle is passed through the clear corneal paracentesis and into the tip of the hollow 26-gauge needle. Both of these are withdrawn externally from the sclera. The 26-gauge needle is again placed through the scleral fixation site a millimeter away from the first pass. At this time, an iris spatula or hook can be used to elevate the malpositioned IOL up to the iris plane. The tip of the hollow needle is passed beneath the free-floating haptic and then above the optic to meet with the other end of the polypropylene suture that has been placed through the same corneal paracentesis as the first. This needle is brought out through the sclera as tension is applied to the other side of the suture to secure the haptic. The suture knot is rotated into the sclera. Visualization can be dramatically improved with the placement of 2 nylon iris retractors through the peripheral clear cornea in the region of refixation.

References

1. Masket S, Osher RH. Late complications with intraocular lens dislocation after capsulorrhexis in pseudoexfoliation syndrome. *J Cataract Refract Surg.* 2002; 28:1481-1484.
2. Siepser SB. The closed chamber slipping suture technique for iris repair. *Ann Ophthalmol.* 1994;26(3): 71-72.
3. Chang DF. Siepser slipknot for McCannel iris-suture fixation of subluxated intraocular lenses. *J Cataract Refract Surg.* 2004;30:1170-1176.
4. Condon GP. Peripheral iris fixation of a foldable acrylic posterior chamber intraocular lens in the absence of capsule support. *Techniques in Ophthalmology.* 2004;2:104-109.

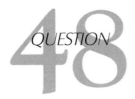
How Do I Explant
an Intraocular Lens
6 Months Following Surgery?

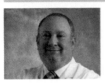

Stephen Lane, MD

Reasons for explantation of an intraocular lens (IOL) are variable and include disloca-tion/decentration, incorrect IOL power, glare/optical aberrations, calcification, and other (IOL damage, uveitis-glaucoma-hyphema syndrome [UGH], retinal detachment [RD], infectious cystoid macular edema [CME]) operative complications (Table 48-1).

General principles for IOL explantation can be divided into preoperative and intraop-erative considerations.

Preoperative Considerations

Explantation of an IOL demands that the surgeon is knowledgeable about the style and characteristics of the IOL that is to be explanted. In this way, formulation of a surgi-cal plan can be made that would include the use of special instrumentation, equipment, IOLs, and institution of surgical techniques that are necessary to maximize results and minimize complications. For example, if an eyelet is present on the IOL haptic, chances are high that fibrosis to the capsular bag is present and attempts to rotate the IOL dur-ing explantation could cause zonular compromise. Therefore, if excessive resistance during removal is met, consideration for cutting the haptic and leaving it rather than attempting complete removal might be entertained earlier in the course of the procedure. Additionally, an alternate plan can be prepared in the event of a broken or torn capsule or zonular dehiscence, including the need for automated vitrectomy.

Table 48-1

Rank Order of Etiologies of Intraocular Lens Explantation Dislocation/Decentration

- Incorrect IOL power
- Glare/optical aberrations
- Calcification
- Other (IOL damage, UGH, RD, infectious, CME, operative complications)

Adapted from Mamalis N, Davis B, Nilson CD, Hickman MS, Leboyer RM. Complications of foldable intraocular lenses requiring explantation or secondary intervention—2003 survey update. *J Cataract Refract Surg.* 2004;30(10):2209-2218.

Intraoperative Considerations

The use of local or general anesthesia is usually recommended to afford maximal patient comfort since frequently significant intraocular manipulation is necessary. The surgeon should have a variety of microhooks, scissors, and ophthalmic viscosurgical devices (OVDs) available. Additionally, bimanual irrigation and aspiration (I&A) and vitrectomy are not only helpful but often necessary. Surgical manipulations should be carried out within a closed system as much as possible. This usually begins by performing a single paracentesis or paired paracenteses (about 180 degrees apart if paired). Next, after finding or creating a space between the IOL and the anterior capsule (often found at the haptic-optic junction), injection of a dispersive OVD through one of the paracenteses is performed, thereby "viscodissecting" the IOL free from the capsule. If the anterior capsule is adherent for 360 degrees onto the IOL surface, a 30-gauge needle on a tuberculin syringe is helpful to undermine the capsular edge, giving adequate space to initiate OVD viscodissection. Care must be taken to avoid overinflation of the bag with OVD as the bag is dissected open. Once the capsular bag is inflated open, attempts to rotate the IOL are made using Sinsky, Kuglen, or equivalent hooks. If the lens has been adequately dissected free from the capsule, it should rotate easily. Next, using a bimanual approach (either through both paracenteses or through the wound and a paracentesis), the IOL can be rotated out of the capsular bag into the anterior chamber with the dispersive OVD protecting the endothelium and other intraocular structures. Iris/capsule retraction with a single hook while rotating the IOL with another hook allows for adequate visualization and also acts as a fulcrum against the haptic of a multipiece IOL, which aids in ushering the IOL into the anterior segment.

Removal of the IOL from the anterior chamber will depend on the IOL style and the wound size desired by the surgeon. Enlarging the wound to 6 mm or more allows direct removal of most IOLs regardless of style. However, sutures are likely to be required to close the operative wound. If the desired wound size is 3 mm or less, other techniques are required.[1,2]

MULTIPIECE SILICONE INTRAOCULAR LENSES

Cutting the IOL in half (bisecting the optic) within the anterior chamber with microscissors can be performed in most cases under OVD control. Cohesive OVDs are helpful in maintaining the anterior chamber space during manipulations in IOL removal. Scissor types to perform these cutting maneuvers may be vertical acting (ie, Rappazzo haptic scissors or Grieshaber scissors) or more conventional horizontal acting scissors (ie, modified Wescott or Vannas scissors). IOL explantation systems have also been devised that include special scissors and holding forceps. The holding forceps can be particularly helpful with silicone IOLs, which tend to be quite slippery, necessitating stabilization while they are being cut. To avoid the need to remove 2 pieces (when the IOL is completely bisected), the optic can be incompletely bisected, leaving a hinge with approximately one-eighth of the optic diameter uncut. In this technique, as the optic is grasped and externalization is initiated, the optic becomes elongated and can be removed in one piece through a 3-mm to 4-mm incision. Similarly, a quadrant of the optic can be cut from the optic and removed. The remaining three-quarters portion of the lens optic is then rotated out of the eye.

SINGLE-PIECE SILICONE INTRAOCULAR LENSES

As with multipiece silicone IOLs, single-piece silicone IOLs are most easily removed from the anterior chamber by completely bisecting the optic and removing the 2 pieces individually. Use of an intraocular snare can also be helpful in these cases.

HYDROPHOBIC ACRYLIC INTRAOCULAR LENSES

Most hydrophobic acrylic IOLs can be cut and manipulated in a fashion similar to those discussed above with silicone IOLs. They are of course much more difficult to cut given their different biomechanical properties. However, unlike silicone IOLs, hydrophobic acrylic IOLs may often be folded in half under OVD control within the anterior chamber. By inserting a cyclodialysis spatula through a paracentesis 180 degrees away from the main incision site and under the IOL optic, a folding forceps is placed through the main incision site over the IOL optic. Closing the IOL forceps over the spatula forces the IOL optic to fold in half after which the spatula and IOL/folding forceps are removed from the eye. After placement of the new foldable IOL through the unenlarged 3-mm to 4-mm incision, bimanual I&A can be used to remove residual cortex and OVD in a controlled fashion, maintaining a closed system.

Presence of Open Posterior Capsule

If the posterior capsule is open, removal of an IOL is significantly more complicated and challenging. Attempts to rotate the IOL within the capsular bag may be impossible because of the inability of the OVD to adequately viscodissect the IOL free from the capsular periphery as it instead escapes posteriorly through the opening in the posterior capsule. As a result, the capsule may need to be sacrificed during the IOL explantation process. The explanting surgeon must be prepared to perform a limbal or pars plana vitrectomy in the presence of an open posterior capsule because vitreous presentation is likely. In the absence of a posterior capsule, the surgeon must be prepared to implant an anterior chamber IOL or suture an IOL to the iris or sclera.

References

1. Osher RH. *Video Journal of Cataract and Refractive Surgery.* 2000;XVI(1).
2. Osher RH, Cionni RJ, Foster RE, Blumenkrantz MS, Da Mata AP. Surgical repositioning and explantation of intraocular lens. In: Steinert RF, ed. *Cataract Surgery.* Philadelphia: WB Saunders; 2004.

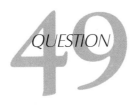

MY PSEUDOEXFOLIATION PATIENT HAS NEWLY DISCOVERED PSEUDOPHACODONESIS 5 YEARS FOLLOWING SURGERY. HOW SHOULD I PROCEED?

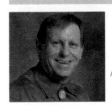

Alan S. Crandall, MD

Pseudoexfoliation syndrome[1] is a relatively common systemic disorder (up to 35% of patients over the age of 70) with well-known ocular sequelae. There is deposition of an ancillary fibrillary substance on all structures of the anterior chamber. Of course, pseudoexfoliation is highly associated with glaucoma and with complications during cataract extractions.[2,3] The iris involvement may lead to poor pupil dilation, which further increases the risk for cataract surgery complications. The accumulation of pseudoexfoliation material is associated with a proteolytic process that probably leads to decreased tensile strength in the zonules.[4] The capsule is also more brittle in pseudoexfoliation syndrome. Fortunately, with modern phacoemulsification techniques such as continuous curvilinear capsulorrhexis, chopping, and the use of capsular tension rings (CTRs) or capsule retractors, the surgical complication rate in these eyes has dropped dramatically.[5]

Late spontaneous dislocation of the entire intraocular lens (IOL) and bag complex in pseudoexfoliation was reported relatively recently.[6] The dislocation may occur 2 months to 17 years postoperatively while the average is approximately 8.5 years after surgery. In our original report, most of the IOLs were made of polymethylmethacrylate (PMMA). Since that report, we have had more than 100 additional cases involving the entire gamut of IOL styles and materials, from single-piece silicone to 3-piece acrylics. To date, Nick

Figure 49-1. Placement of the haptic fixation with a 9-0 prolene suture.

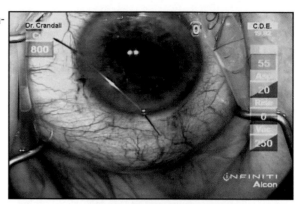

Figure 49-2. Double-armed 10-0 polypropylene suture to fixate each haptic to the peripheral iris with a modified McCannel suture.

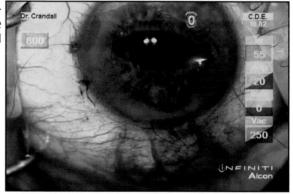

Mamalis, and myself, as well as other investigators, have been unable to identify any risk factors other than the pseudoexfoliation to explain the late dislocation. The true incidence is unknown but is probably quite low. Therefore, I do not believe that any major change in surgical technique is advocated. We did not see this situation prior to continuous curvilinear capsulorrhexis with phacoemulsification, but the reduction in surgical complications allowing for capsular bag fixation may be enough to explain the situation.

Most patients do not present to the ophthalmologist until the entire bag-IOL complex has completely dislocated. However, some patients may note fluctuating vision and can present with pseudophacodonesis and minimal subluxation. Surgical management is certainly easier the earlier the patient presents.

Surgical management of the bag-IOL dislocation depends on the type of IOL. The dislocated bag-IOL can be explanted and, following an anterior vitrectomy, replaced with an anterior chamber IOL. There is no other choice but to do this for a silicone plate haptic IOL. However, IOLs with loop haptics can be suture fixated to either the sclera or to the iris, and this is my preference. A double-armed 9-0 polypropylene suture (Figure 49-1) can sclerally fixate each haptic by first ensnaring it with a lasso technique. One needle is passed through the bag and underneath the haptic before exiting through the ciliary sulcus. The second needle passes over the haptic before exiting alongside the first pass.

The technique I prefer is to first bring the complex up to the pupillary plane,[7] where vitreous and the surrounding capsular remnants are removed with a vitrectomy handpiece. I then use a double-armed 10-0 polypropylene suture to fixate each haptic to the peripheral iris with a modified McCannel suture (Figure 49-2).

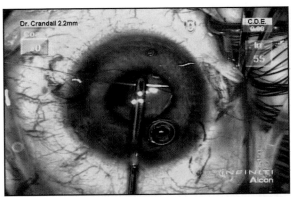

Figure 49-3. Scleral fixation of the lens with a CTR.

As a possible preventive measure, some surgeons advocate making a relaxing cut in the capsulorrhexis margin after the IOL has been implanted. Alternatively, this can be done postoperatively with the YAG laser. These strategies have not been tested by a randomized study and because this is such a late postoperative complication, it will take a long time to prove whether any preventive measure is effective. Others feel that implanting a CTR may help by more evenly redistributing and resisting capsular contractile forces (Figure 49-3). Although CTRs may help prevent capsule contraction, if bag dislocation is due to progressive zonular weakness, they probably will not stop the process. One advantage of having a CTR in the bag would be that it could be used to sclerally fixate the complex. A final option is to use a modified CTR, such as a Cionni I or II, which has an eyelet that can be used for scleral suture fixation.[8] However, Miyake camera views in cadaver eyes show that inserting these can cause significant iatrogenic damage to the zonules.[9] Because the incidence of late bag-IOL dislocation is probably low, one must carefully weigh the risks of inserting these devices against the theoretical benefit.

Conclusion

Late dislocation of the entire bag-IOL complex in pseudoexfoliation is unusual but not rare. Careful follow-up of pseudoexfoliation patients postoperatively is important and may afford an earlier opportunity for corrective surgery (Figure 49-4). Recommendations include making a capsulorrhexis that is relatively large (5.5 mm) and promptly treating any capsular phimosis with YAG laser relaxing cuts. Whether to routinely implant a CTR in every pseudoexfoliation patient is controversial and is probably not necessary.

References

1. Naumann GOH, Schlotzer-Schrehardt U, Kuchie M. Pseudoexfoliation syndrome for the comprehensive ophthalmologist: intraocular and systemic manifestations [review]. *Ophthalmology.* 1998;105:951-968.
2. Avramides S, Traianidis P, Sakkias G. Cataract surgery lens implantation in eyes with exfoliation syndrome. *J Cataract Refract Surg.* 1997;23:583-587.
3. Bartholomew RS. Lens displacement associated with pseudo capsular exfoliation: a report on 19 cases in the Southern Bantu. *Br J Ophthalmol.* 1970;54:744-750.
4. Skuta GL, Parrish RK 2nd, Hodapp E, et al. Zonular dialysis during extracapsular cataract extraction in pseudoexfoliation syndrome. *Arch Ophthalmol.* 1987;105:632-634.

Figure 49-4. Postoperative results.

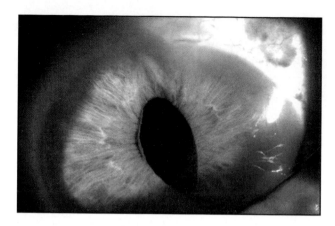

5. Fine IH, Hoffman RS. Phacoemulsification in the presence of pseudoexfoliation: challenges and options. *J Cataract Refract Surg.* 1997;23:160-165.
6. Jehan FS, Mamalis N, Crandall AS. Spontaneous late dislocation of intraocular lens within the capsular bag in pseudoexfoliation patients. *Ophthalmology.* 2001;108(10):1727-1731.
7. Chang DF. Viscoelastic levitation of posteriorly dislocated IOLs from the anterior vitreous. *J Cataract Refract Surg.* 2002;28:1515-1519.
8. Cionni RJ, Osher RH. Management of profound zonular dialysis or weakness with a new endocapsular ring designed for scleral fixation. *J Cataract Refract Surg.* 1998;24:1299-1306.
9. Ahmed II, Cionni RJ, Kranemann C, Crandall AS. Optimal timing of capsular tension ring implantation: Miyake-Apple video analysis. *J Cataract Refract Surg.* 2005;31(9):1809-1813.

Financial Disclosures

QUESTION 1

Douglas D. Koch, MD has no conflicts to disclose for this material.

QUESTION 2

Walter J. Stark, MD has no financial relationship to disclose.

QUESTION 3

Bradford J. Shingleton, MD has research support from Alcon, Allergan, and Pfizer. He is a consultant for Bausch & Lomb and iScience. These have no relation to anything in the chapter.

QUESTION 4

Thomas Samuelson, MD has no financial relationship to disclose for this subject.

QUESTION 5

Richard J. Mackool, MD is a consultant for Alcon and Impex.

QUESTION 6

Bonnie An Henderson, MD is on the speaker's bureau at Alcon, but has no financial interest in the material presented.

QUESTION 7

Francis W. Price, Jr, MD is a consultant for Alcon Laboratories; Allergan, Inc; IntraLase Corporation; OPHTEC; LUX Biosciences; and Surgical Specialities. He is an equity owner of Calhoun Vision. He receives lecture fees from Alcon Laboratories; Allergan, Inc; IntraLase Corporation; Moria; and OPHTEC.

QUESTION 8

Jack T. Holladay, MD, MSEE, FACS is a consultant for Advanced Medical Optics and NIDEK.

QUESTION 9

Warren E. Hill, MD, FACS is a consultant for Alcon Laboratories and Carl Zeiss Meditec.

QUESTION 10

Paul Koch, MD has no conflicts to disclose for this chapter.

QUESTION 11

Kerry D. Solomon, MD has financial relationships with Alcon, Allergan, Advanced Medical Optics, and Bausch & Lomb.

QUESTION 12

R. Bruce Wallace III, MD, FACS is a consultant for Allergan, Inc and Advanced Medical Optics, Inc.

QUESTION 13

Francis S. Mah, MD receives research support from and is a consultant for Alcon Labs, Inc; Allergan, Inc; Insite, Inc; Polymedix, Inc; and MPEX, Inc.

QUESTION 14

Kenneth J. Rosenthal, MD, FACS has no conflicts for this chapter.

QUESTION 15

Randall J. Olson, MD has no financial relationships that are relevant to his article, but he is a paid consultant for Allergan, Advanced Medical Optics, and BD. He also has a financial interest in Chakshu and Calhoun Vision.

QUESTION 16

Johnny Gayton, MD is on the speaker's bureaus at Alcon and Allergan.

QUESTION 17

Rosa Braga-Mele, MEd, MD, FRCSC has no financial interest to disclose related to this chapter.

QUESTION 18

William J. Fishkind, MD, FACS is a paid consultant for Advanced Medical Optics, receives a royalty income from Thieme Publishers, and is a lecturer for Bausch & Lomb.

QUESTION 19

I. Howard Fine, MD is a consultant for Advanced Medical Optics, Inc; Bausch & Lomb, Inc; iScience, Inc; Carl Zeiss Meditec, Inc; and Omeros Corporation. He also receives research and travel support from Alcon Laboratories, Inc; Eyeonics, Inc; STAAR Surgical, Inc; and Rayner, Ltd.

QUESTION 20

Robert H. Osher, MD is a consultant for Alcon and Advanced Medical Optics.

QUESTION 21

Terry Kim, MD is a consultant for Alcon, Allergan, ISTA, Becton-Dickinson Ophthalmics, and Hyperbranch Medical Technology. He receives grant support from Alcon and Allergan. He is on the speaker's bureau at Alcon, Allergan, Bausch & Lomb, and ISTA.

QUESTION 22

Robert J. Cionni, MD has financial relationships with Alcon Laboratories and Morcher GmBh.

QUESTION 23

Samuel F. Masket, MD is a consultant for Alcon, Visiogen, PowerVision, Othera, and Omeros. He is on the speaker's bureau at Alcon.

QUESTION 24

Steve A. Arshinoff, MD, FRCSC is a consultant for Alcon Laboratories and Advanced Medical Optics.

QUESTION 25

David F. Chang, MD is a consultant for Advanced Medical Optics, Alcon, and Visiogen.

QUESTION 26

Roger F. Steinert, MD has no relevant financial relationships.

QUESTION 27

Barry S. Seibel, MD is a consultant for Bausch & Lomb Surgical. He also receives a royalty from SLACK Incorporated for his text, *Phacodynamics: Mastering the Tools and Techniques of Phacoemulsification Surgery, Fourth Edition.*

QUESTION 28

Lisa B. Arbisser, MD has ad hoc honoraria and research grants from Alcon and Advanced Medical Optics and has been a speaker for Alcon in the last year.

QUESTION 29

Iqbal Ike K. Ahmed, MD, FRCSC receives research grant/support from Alcon, Allergan, Aquesys, Carl Zeiss Meditec, iScience, Pfizer, SOLX, and Visiogen. He receives speakers honoraria from Alcon, Advanced Medical Optics, Allergan, Carl Zeiss Meditec, and SOLX. He is a consultant and receives consulting fees from Alcon, Advanced Medical Optics, Aquesys, Carl Zeiss Meditec, Clarity Medical Systems, Coronado, Eyelight, Pfizer, SOLX, and Transcend Medical.

Question 30

Howard V. Gimbel, MD, MPH, FRCSC, FACS has no financial relationship to disclose.

Question 31

Louis D. "Skip" Nichamin, MD has no financial relationship to disclose.

Question 32

Scott E. Burk, MD, PhD has no financial relationship to disclose.

Question 33

Thomas A. Oetting, MS, MD has no financial relationship to disclose.

Question 34

Elizabeth A. Davis, MD, FACS is a consultant for Advanced Medical Optics, Bausch & Lomb, Intralase, and STAAR Surgical. She is on the speaker's bureaus at ISTA, Allergan, and Refractec. However, with respect to the article she wrote, she has no conflicts.

Question 35

Manus C. Kraff, MD has no financial relationship to disclose.

Question 36

Eric D. Donnenfeld, MD is a consultant for Allergan, Advanced Medical Optics, Alcon, Bausch & Lomb, TLC Laser Centers, and Eyeimaginations.

Question 37

James P. Gills, MD has no financial relationship to disclose.

Question 38

Richard A. Lewis, MD has no financial relationship to disclose.

Question 39

Luther L. Fry, MD has no financial relationship to disclose.

Question 40

Nick Mamalis, MD performs contract research for Alcon, Advanced Medical Optics, Allergan, Bausch & Lomb, and Calhoun and is on the scientific advisory boards of Medennium and Visiogen.

Question 41

Michael B. Raizman, MD has no financial relationships to disclose for this chapter.

QUESTION 42

Stanley Chang, MD is on the speaker's bureau at Alcon Surgical.

QUESTION 43

Mark Packer, MD is a consultant for Advanced Medical Optics, Inc; Advanced Vision Science, Inc; Bausch & Lomb, Inc; Carl Zeiss Meditec, Inc; Carl Zeiss Surgical GmbH; Celgene Corporation; Ethicon, Inc; Gerson Lehman Group, Inc; iScience Surgical Corporation; Johnson & Johnson Vision Care, Inc (Vistakon Division); Leerink Swann & Company; Medtronic Xomed, Inc; Visiogen, Inc; and VisionCare, Inc. He also has travel, research, and honoraria from Alcon Laboratories, Inc; Endo Optiks, Inc; eyeonics, inc; and STAAR Surgical, Inc.

QUESTION 44

Kevin M. Miller, MD has no relevant financial relationships to disclose for this material.

QUESTION 45

Kevin L. Waltz, OD, MD is a consultant for Advanced Medical Optics and eyeonics.

QUESTION 46

Richard L. Lindstrom, MD has financial relationships with Advanced Medical Optics, Bausch & Lomb, Alcon, eyeonics, and Santen.

QUESTION 47

Garry P. Condon, MD is on the speaker's bureau at Alcon, Merck, and Pfizer.

QUESTION 48

Stephen Lane, MD has financial relationships with Alcon, Bausch & Lomb, VisionCare, Visiogen, and WaveTech.

QUESTION 49

Alan S. Crandall, MD is a consultant and on the speaker's bureau at Alcon; on the speaker's bureau at Allergan and Pfizer; on the advisory board at I-Science; iSportgames, Inc; eSinomed; Omeros; and *Glaucoma Today;* and on the editorial board at *Ocular Surgery News.*

INDEX